PENG

THE DI

Ishi Khosla is a practising clinical nutritionist, consultant, writer, researcher and an entrepreneur.

She is actively involved in clinical practice at the Centre for Dietary Counseling in Delhi, where she deals with a wide range of nutrition-related health problems including obesity, cardiovascular disease, diabetes, gastrointestinal problems, allergies, etc. She has recently developed the first fully Web-based weight-management programme in India: www.theweightmonitor.com. Passionate about nutrition and a strong believer in the power of foods, she has spearheaded a path-breaking health food company, Whole Foods India, which produces health foods and operates health cafes.

She is a consultant to several organizations and is also a board member of Lady Irwin College, University of Delhi. She lectures extensively, is invited frequently to radio and television programmes and also contributes regularly to some of the country's most respected publications. She has written two other books, most recently *Is Wheat Killing You?*, also published by Penguin Books.

As part of her commitment towards community nutrition and public health, Ms Khosla founded the Celiac Society for Delhi, the first of its kind in India, to spread awareness about coeliac disease, a condition caused by gluten intolerance. She has been conferred with several awards and recognitions in her field and has also been listed among the twenty-five most powerful women in the country by the India Today Group.

ishi khosla

the diet doctor

the scientifically proven way to lose weight

PENGUIN BOOKS

PENGUIN BOOKS

USA | Canada | UK | Ireland | Australia
New Zealand | India | South Africa | China

Penguin Books is part of the Penguin Random House group of companies whose addresses can be found at global.penguinrandomhouse.com

Published by Penguin Random House India Pvt. Ltd
7th Floor, Infinity Tower C, DLF Cyber City,
Gurgaon 122 002, Haryana, India

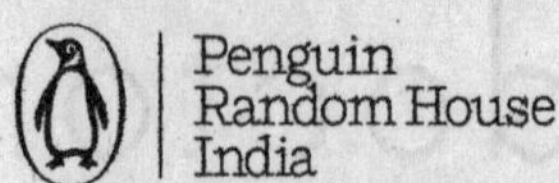

First published by Penguin Books India 2013

10 9 8 7 6 5 4 3 2

While every effort has been made to verify the authenticity of the information contained in this book, the publisher and the author are in no way liable for the use of the information contained in this book.

ISBN 9780143064930

Typeset in Requiem (OTF) by R. Ajith Kumar, New Delhi
Printed at Repro Knowledgecast Limited, Thane

www.penguinbooksindia.com

I dedicate this book to all those who have impacted my life.

My father, who always knew butter was better than margarine,
and my mother, who taught me biology like a story.

My in-laws for their affection and constant support.

My husband and my children for their unconditional love.

CONTENTS

INTRODUCTION

I must start with a confession—what started out to be a book on nutrition, with a chapter on obesity management, turned out to be something quite different. As a nutritionist, I believe that adopting principles of healthy eating along with common sense is all that it takes to keep the extra kilos off. But somewhere down the road I realized that this area needs undivided attention.

Most of my clients had, prior to our interaction, followed diets and visited dieticians who gave them diet charts, which they would follow blindly. Diets were based on self-styled theories and had been made into mysteries. Often, most of these theories had little scientific basis and would invariably be hard to practise in the real world in a sustained way. My efforts towards convincing my clients that they could continue eating the way they do with simple modifications and still lose weight were received with scepticism initially. In no time, however, things changed. Scepticism changed to empowerment and confidence and I began to see how more and more clients were transforming their lives. Even now I am often asked as to what diet I prescribe. Short of a name, I simply say that it is a 'scientifically based healthy diet'. This 'nameless' and simple diet has always been all about arming my clients with the right information so that they can design their own healthy-eating plans, suitable for their specific needs.

The Diet Doctor takes you through all the phases of your weight-loss journey and gives you all the information a sound nutritionist would use to assess your case and plan a diet for you. My philosophy is to help you understand foods and their effects on your body, and then train you to move towards healthy eating. So you will get a lot of science here, all made extremely accessible. The first step to planning your diet is to really know the facts and this book gives you everything you need to know. I've also discussed ideas such as motivations, the way society works and how most people eat, so that you may gain awareness of your eating patterns and the ability to control them.

Most of my clients are extremely busy so what they really want from me is a fixed plan that they can follow, and you might be like them. But understanding these issues so you won't get misled any more is worthwhile. The key to my 'no-diet diet' is to help you incorporate healthy-eating principles into your life for ever. Nor do I believe in quick fixes. Healthy weight loss needs to be steady and slow—ideally 1–½ kg per week—and although I have given you a diet plan for faster weight loss, I urge you to use that only if absolutely necessary.

Looking at me today, most people are surprised to find that the reason behind my choosing my career path is rooted in my own weight problem during childhood. An obese child, still called 'Fatty' by my cousins, I often ate breakfast twice and was always ready for good food. I would wait for my mother to put a chunk of white butter, which she churned in our kitchen regularly, on my parathas every day. Our home was all about delicious food. Home-made ice creams, breads, pizzas, cakes, cookies, desserts, jams, jellies, pickles, rasgullas, rasmalai, samosas, chaat, potato wafers—we had it all.

At the same time there was a scientific atmosphere within the house. My father was a chemistry specialist and my mother a home scientist, so terms like 'trans-fatty acids', 'melting points', 'freezing points' and 'coal-tar dyes' were used regularly. It was not surprising that I absorbed this knowledge along the way and became hugely interested in food. I took to baking when I was just 8 and started documenting my recipes when I was all of 12 years.

By then, I had started to become aware of my excess weight subconsciously and had started counting calories. My cousins and I became completely obsessed—calculating the amount we ate and how much we burnt. If we ate more, we jogged extra. Within a year, I had lost all my excess weight and began to be called 'Thinny-Pinny' by my English teacher. It was then that I dropped the idea of doing medicine and decided to focus on nutrition. I joined Lady Irwin College and eventually completed my master's in foods and nutrition. Soon after, I got married and some years later joined the Escorts Heart Institute and Research Centre as Head of Nutrition in the Department of Preventive Cardiology. During my years of practice there, I felt the need to make a difference to people's lives and eating habits rather than giving out diet charts. I could not see myself reducing this absolutely fascinating field to mere calorie counting—there was so much more to it. My desire to practise more meaningfully led to the birth of my health food company, Whole Foods India, and my own practice at the Centre for Dietary Counseling. This book is a compilation of my learning through these years. Happy reading.

Table of measurements

1 cup	=	200 mg/200 ml
1 tbsp	=	15 mg/15 ml
1 tsp	=	5 mg/5 ml
A pinch	=	¼ tsp
A handful	=	30 gm

A standard cup

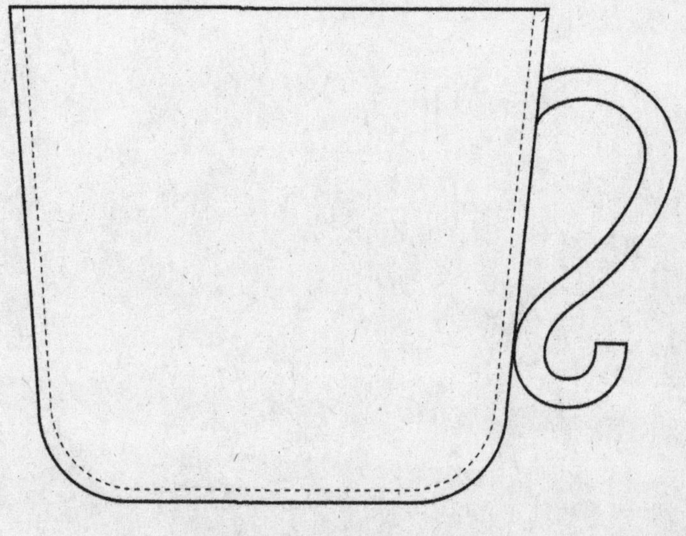

2.6 inches in height
3 inches in diameter

(drawn to scale)

1

HOW FAT IS FAT?

> ## ✚ THE DOCTOR SAYS
>
> With nearly half the Indian population being obese (according to the Asia Pacific Criteria of Obesity issued by the World Health Organization [WHO]), the battle of the bulge is getting as challenging as the war on terrorism. Obesity comes with huge baggage, both for the individual and community. It has massive implications for your health. Don't listen to articles and TV shows that tell you that you should accept your body the way it is. It is never OK to do so. In this chapter we look at exactly what being overweight does to you and discuss how to assess your weight as scientifically and accurately as possible.

Weight and diseases

Obesity markedly increases the risk of heart disease, type 2 diabetes, metabolic syndrome (see section on metabolic obesity, p. 14) and hypertension. People with obesity have double the risk of heart disease and stroke and more than triple the risk of diabetes, compared to those who are of normal weight. A weight gain of 5–10 kg over your ideal body weight (IBW) increases your chances of developing type 2 diabetes; such individuals are twice as vulnerable as those who have not gained weight. The prevalence of fatty liver, degenerative arthritis, kidney and gall bladder stones, erectile dysfunction, gout, varicose veins, chronic inflammation, reduced sleep and sleep apnoea increases in proportion to the degree of excess weight. For every kg increase in weight above the IBW, the risk of developing arthritis increases by 9–13 per cent.

Obesity increases the risk of some types of cancer—endometrial, colon, gall bladder, prostate and post-menopausal breast cancer. It has been reported that obesity increases the risk of breast cancer in post-menopausal women by 50 per cent and women who gain more than 10 kg from age 18 to midlife double their risk of developing post-menopausal breast cancer. Some studies suggest that gaining as little as 2 kg at the age of 50 or later can increase the risk of breast cancer by 30 per cent. In addition, childhood obesity too has recently been linked to cancer.

Being overweight increases the risk of early puberty, polycystic ovaries, irregular menstrual cycles, infertility and complications in pregnancy like gestational diabetes, stillbirths, birth defects, large babies, and low levels of testosterone and breast development in boys. Obesity also increases the risk of poor gastrointestinal health, hyperacidity, gastroesophageal reflux disease (GERD), irritable bowel syndrome and constipation. Paradoxically, obesity is also associated with malnutrition and common nutritional deficiencies, which include iron, calcium and vitamins, particularly vitamins A and D.

Other complications include poor skin and hair health (acne, darkening of skin, hair fall, dandruff, brittle nails, fungal infections, athlete's foot, etc.), depressed immune system, autoimmune disorders, allergies and sinusitis, poor bone health (osteoporosis/osteopenia), bow legs, difficulty in walking, pain or stiffness in knees and hips, easy fractures, poor self-esteem, anxiety, mood swings, depression, stress and fatigue. In short, obesity reduces the quality of life for almost anyone it affects.

Besides these, the economic burden to the individual or the nation cannot be ignored. Huge percentages of the gross domestic product (GDP) are being spent on health care along with the loss of productivity due to obesity-related diseases. Research in the US indicates that medical bills on account of ill health due to obesity amounted to US$51.6 billion and led to a loss of productivity worth US$3.9 billion. Not surprisingly, obese workers are twice as likely to miss work. In China and India, lost productivity due to diet-related diseases amounted to 0.5 per cent and 0.7 per cent of the GDP respectively in 2001.[1] Statistics indicate that the rate at which the number of people suffering from being overweight has increased is alarming, especially in 'nations in transition' like ours. **Obesity has been declared one of the top ten risk conditions in the world and one of the top five in the developed world by the WHO**. Have I scared you enough? Well, the good news is that all of us can lose weight and become fit if we want to.

Many of you will have bought this book because you want to lose weight to look good or shed those extra kilos before an important event. That's all right but remember that losing weight should not just be about looking good but also about being fit and feeling good about yourself, physically, mentally and spiritually. **Simply said, keeping your body at its optimum weight (or close to it) is a health must and non-negotiable**. I have had clients with very extreme cases of obesity who are now well on their way to fitness. And you can be too. The first step is to figure out exactly how much weight you need to lose, followed

1 Christopher Wanjek, 'The History and Economics of Workplace Nutrition' in *Food at Work: Workplace Solutions for Malnutrition, Obesity and Chronic Diseases* (Geneva: Publications Bureau, International Labour Office, 2005), 12.

by losing that weight gradually so you reach your ideal weight/size and shape the right way.

Discover your optimum weight

Your weight as shown by the weighing scale may not be the real indicator of the levels of your body fat and fitness. Some indices have been established to assess your ideal weight, the distribution of fat in your body, and body shape which help predict your risk of developing certain diseases. To get an accurate measure of what you need to lose and your levels of fitness, the following are useful:

1. Body mass index (BMI)
2. Total body fat percentage and distribution
3. Waist circumference
4. Waist-to-height ratio (WHtR)
5. Body shape

Body mass index (BMI)

BMI is the most basic measure of obesity and is the internationally accepted standard of measuring how overweight you are. It is calculated using your weight (in kilograms) and height (in square metres), and is independent of gender and age. It also helps to identify individuals who are at risk of developing associated complications. As the BMI increases, the risk of developing associated conditions, such as type 2 diabetes mellitus, heart disease, stroke, gall bladder disease, osteoarthritis, sleep apnoea and cancer, also increases. However, it must be clear that the relation between BMI and health risks varies among different people and populations.

Three easy steps to calculate your BMI:

1. Check your weight on the weighing scale. Calculate your weight in kilograms.
2. Check your height on the height scale. Calculate your height in square metres.
3. Calculate your BMI by dividing weight in kilograms by height in square metres.

BMI = weight (kg)/height (m^2)

Table 1.1: Relationship between BMI and disease risk

Status	BMI (kg/m^2)	Disease risk
Underweight	<18.5	
Normal	18.5–22.9	Increasing but acceptable risk
Overweight	23.0–24.9	Increased risk
Obesity I	25.0–29.9	High risk
Obesity II	≥30.0	Higher risk

Source: Data from Robert C. Weisell, 'Body Mass Index as an Indicator of Obesity', *Asia Pacific Journal of Clinical Nutrition* 11, no. 8 (December 2008): S2681–84.

BMI, however, has limitations. It can neither help distinguish the pattern of obesity, nor can it help differentiate between fat and muscle mass. Some people with an 'obese' BMI might have a normal body fat percentage and higher muscle mass, while others with a normal BMI might have excess fat and reduced muscle mass. For example, athletes tend to have a high BMI even if they are not fat and individuals shorter than 5 feet also have a high BMI despite not being overweight.

For a given BMI, women have more fat than men. This is also true for Asians as compared to Caucasians and blacks. At a given BMI, Indians/Asians have about 5 per cent higher body fat than other populations. This is usually because Asians have a smaller body frame and a genetic predisposition towards excess body fat. For this reason, Asians with a BMI of more than 23 are considered overweight while those with a BMI of 27 and above are considered obese.

Total percentage and distribution of body fat

Fat behaves differently on different parts of the body, and the location of fat is more important than its amount in a given individual. For example, you might have low body fat overall but excess fat on your belly. This fat is usually more dangerous than fat in other areas as it increases your vulnerability to heart disease and diabetes. Researchers tracked a group of patients who went through liposuction surgery on arms, legs and thighs to get rid of flab from the body. They found no improvement in blood pressure, triglyceride levels, glucose tolerance or cholesterol profiles.[2] This is because the fat around your liver, kidney and intestines, also called visceral fat, is different from subcutaneous fat, which is right under the skin. Subcutaneous fat is easier to lose than visceral fat, and visceral fat is what causes most of our health problems. In terms of the impact on our health, the amount of fat our body carries is less important than where our body stores it.

The indices that help identify the location of fat include waist circumference, waist-to-height ratio and body shape. The most

2 S. Klein and others, 'Absence of an Effect of Liposuction on Insulin Action and Risk Factors for Coronary Heart Disease', *The New England Journal of Medicine* 350, no. 25 (June 2004): 2549–57.

accurate way to determine how much fat you are carrying and where is to go through a body fat or body composition analysis or estimation done through a machine.

Table 1.2: Optimum levels of fat

Category	Optimum levels of fat
Men	12–20 per cent
Women	20–25 per cent
Athletes (both sexes)	7–10 per cent

Waist circumference

Generally, your waist refers to the thinnest part of your upper body or trunk. But for this measurement your waist is measured at the maximum part of your trunk. It is an approximate index of intra-abdominal or visceral fat, which is a key factor in obesity-related diseases. Medically, a measurement of less than 80 cm (approximately 31.5 inches) and less than 90 cm (approximately 35.5 inches) is considered acceptable for Indian women and men respectively. Waist circumference as an index has been found particularly useful for individuals who have a normal BMI but a large waist circumference; it is an indicator of increased risk of type 2 diabetes, abnormal cholesterol levels, high blood pressure, heart disease and other chronic diseases. **Those who are overweight with a larger waist circumference are at a much higher risk of metabolic disorders than those with a waist circumference that falls within the acceptable measurements.** At a given waist size, Indians and other Asians have a higher risk of abnormal cholesterol levels, diabetes and heart disease than Americans and Europeans.

A combined reading of BMI and waist circumference will give you an accurate assessment of your health risks:

1. A high BMI with a low waist circumference may indicate that the BMI is overestimating the severity of obesity and risk of diseases.
2. A low BMI with a high waist circumference may indicate that the BMI is underestimating the severity of obesity and risk of diseases.

The following table is in accordance with WHO-prescribed international standards, and gives the BMI and waist circumference values relevant for populations at large—the information is not just limited to the Asian/Indian population. It explains that disease risk is relative to normal weight and waist circumference. The risk of diseases, especially type 2 diabetes, hypertension and cardiovascular disease, increases significantly with both increased BMI and increased waist circumference.

Table 1.3: Relationship between BMI, waist circumference and disease risk

Status	**BMI (kg/m^2)**	**Obesity class**	**Disease risk**	
			Waist circumference (men <102 cm; women <88 cm)	**Waist circumference (men >102 cm; women >88 cm)**
Underweight	<18.5			
Normal*	18.5–24.9			
Overweight	25.0–29.9		Increased	High

Status	**BMI (kg/m^2)**	**Obesity class**	**Disease risk**	
			Waist circumference (men <102 cm; women <88 cm)	**Waist circumference (men >102 cm; women >88 cm)**
Obesity	30.0–34.9	I	High	Very high
	35.0–35.9	II	Very high	Very high
Extreme Obesity	≥40	III	Extremely high	Extremely high

Source: Data from WHO, 'Obesity: Preventing and Managing the Global Epidemic; Report of a WHO Consultation', *WHO Technical Report Series 894* (2008): i–xii, 1–253.

Note: These BMI values are age independent and the same for both sexes. However, BMI may not correspond to the same degree of fatness in different populations due, in part, to differences in body proportions. The table shows a simplistic relationship between BMI and the risk of co-morbidity, which can be affected by a range of factors including the nature of diet, ethnic group and activity levels.

* Increased waist circumference can be a marker of increased disease risk even for persons of normal weight.

Waist-to-height ratio (WHtR)

A more recent and useful global tool, which is considered relatively more accurate than waist circumference, to measure belly fat is WHtR. Here the calculation is simple: you need to keep your waist circumference at less than half your height. WHtR is a predictor of metabolic syndrome. For example, if your height is 170 cm, your waist circumference should be less than or equal to 85 cm.

Body shape

The simplest way to determine your weight-gain pattern is to look in the mirror. Both men and women gain weight differently and on different parts of the body. If you have a large belly, not much fat on the hips and thin extremities you are likely to be an apple. If, instead, you have a comparatively thinner torso with heavier hips and legs, you're a pear. Apple- and pear-shaped bodies carry different health implications and their weight management too needs to be addressed differently.

Apple

The kind of obesity that results in the apple shape is called abdominal or central obesity. If you have a tendency to gain more weight around your abdomen and waist, your body shape would resemble an apple or an android. This is usually characterized as 'male pattern' obesity. Abdominal fat is linked to higher levels of visceral fat, that is, fat that wraps around your abdomen and internal organs, including the liver, kidneys and pancreas, and promotes inflammation. This type of fat also pushes out your gut, giving you a Buddha belly. It has been found that those who are apple shaped are at a higher risk of developing insulin resistance and chronic conditions including type 2 diabetes, high blood pressure, heart disease, abnormal lipids, abnormal blood clotting, and breast cancer (in women). Most South Asians have a high percentage of body fat and experience a high prevalence of abdominal obesity, associated with even greater health risks.

Pear

The kind of obesity that results in the pear shape is called peripheral obesity. If you have a tendency to gain more weight around your hips and thighs your body shape would resemble a pear or gynoid. This is usually characterized as 'female pattern' obesity. Risks for developing associated conditions are present but are not as high as with those who are apple shaped. The 'apple' with a paunch presents a serious warning of unhealthy blood chemistry and danger ahead.

About half of all the people who have had heart attacks have been found to be suffering from a condition that is referred to by several names—metabolic syndrome, syndrome X, pre-diabetes or insulin resistance. Recognized in 1989 as an entity, it is still being explored and delved into by researchers. In this book, we will refer to it as insulin resistance or metabolic obesity. Unchecked, it can turn into full-blown type 2 diabetes. Widespread among Indians and those with a positive family history of diabetes (that is, with regard to maternal and paternal grandparents, parents or siblings), it can be managed well with diet, exercise and, in some cases, insulin-sensitizing medicines.

Simple and metabolic obesity

Obesity is primarily of two types—simple and metabolic. The way you lose weight differs depending on which category you belong to.

Simple obesity

It is the kind where you gain weight in a generalized fashion. It behaves more predictably—that is, you gain weight gradually, in proportion to excess calories, and lose weight proportionally too. In other words, you lose weight more easily as compared to those with metabolic obesity. People with simple obesity usually do not have a positive family history of diabetes and therefore insulin resistance is not marked.

Metabolic obesity

It is an insulin-resistant state and is much more complex than simple obesity. In your body, the pancreas produces insulin (the blood glucose–regulating hormone) in response to the consumption of carbohydrates, in order to control blood sugar levels. Being insulin resistant means that your body does not respond to the effects of the given amount of insulin the way a normal body should. This is because some of your cells have receptors for insulin which become ineffective. This results in insulin not being able to enter the blood cells to do its job. This means that your pancreas needs to produce more insulin than normal to control your blood sugar levels when you eat carbohydrates (sugar or starch) or consume excessive calories. It results from an excess of insulin in the blood (hyperinsulinemia), and a resistance to its actions. Besides regulating blood sugar levels, insulin also controls your blood fat levels and is a body-building hormone. The higher the level of insulin, the higher is the percentage of fat, particularly in the organs (liver, kidney and spleen), also known as visceral fat. A person with insulin resistance or metabolic obesity experiences a higher insulin secretion compared to a person with simple obesity. For example, if a person with metabolic obesity has a bar of chocolate his body responds by secreting higher insulin compared to a person with simple obesity.

Metabolic obesity is two–three times more common among Indians than simple or general obesity. This is in sharp contrast to whites, who have only a slightly higher rate of metabolic obesity than general obesity, and blacks, who actually have a lower rate of metabolic obesity than simple or general obesity.

Let's contrast two of my clients. Ms A, a severely obese 58-year-old lady, weighed 112 kg at a height of 5 feet 2 inches. Her good dietary compliance along with a little exercise led to a weight loss of 30 kg in less than a year. This averages to 3 kg per month. This is a classic example of simple obesity—she was able to lose a significant amount of weight easily on a disciplined diet. Also, as she doesn't have a family history of diabetes or a history of insulin imbalance, weight loss for her was much easier.

Now take another one of my clients: Ms B is 25 years old and has a strong family history (both paternal and maternal) of diabetes. She has found it very hard to lose weight; in fact, in 3 months she was able to lose just half a kilogram. However, inch loss was significant—she lost 7 cm from the waist, 10 cm from the belly and 6 cm from the hips. Often the phenomenon of losing less weight and more inches is associated with insulin resistance. She is an example of someone suffering from metabolic obesity.

Insulin resistance leads to several health problems. These include abnormal cholesterol levels (high blood triglyceride levels, high low-density lipoprotein [LDL], which is bad cholesterol, and low high-density lipoprotein [HDL], which is good cholesterol), glucose intolerance, high uric acid levels, fatty liver, increased inflammation and clotting tendency of blood, and increased risk of high blood pressure, diabetes mellitus and heart disease. A constellation of these symptoms is sometimes referred to as metabolic syndrome or syndrome X.

Besides abdominal or central obesity, other visible manifestations of metabolic syndrome include darkening and thickening of skin in certain areas (underarms, behind the neck, thigh folds), skin tags, warts, buffalo hump, abnormal breast development in boys, and excessive hair growth in girls and women. Those suffering from insulin resistance also seem to be more prone to inflammatory conditions and lowered immunity. Common manifestations include allergies, asthma, bronchitis, digestive disorders—GERD, hyperacidity, constipation, irritable bowel syndrome—and skin and hair problems including eczema, psoriasis, acne and dandruff.

All obese people, to some degree, are insulin resistant; however, those with a positive family history of type 2 diabetes mellitus tend to be far more severely resistant. It has been shown that polycystic ovarian syndrome (PCOS) in women is also an insulin-resistant state.

It must be remembered that insulin resistance and PCOS are not always easy to identify through blood tests and sonographies. But if you do find it hard to lose weight, and have belly fat, a positive family history of type 2 diabetes, or suffer from any of the three health problems mentioned in association with metabolic syndrome, it might be because you are suffering from insulin resistance or metabolic obesity.

✚ ADDING IT ALL UP

Hopefully this chapter has given you a better understanding of measuring your weight, types of obesity and the risks associated with being overweight or obese. Perhaps one of the newest and most important concepts for you is metabolic obesity or insulin resistance and the constellation of symptoms associated with it. But before we proceed to finding out how to deal with this, exploring as to how and why we gain weight is worthwhile—knowing the problem is half the solution.

2

THE INDIAN CONTEXT

✤ THE DOCTOR SAYS

While people all over the world gain weight for largely the same reasons—quantity and quality of food, lack of physical exercise, stress, specific medical conditions—the Indian body type has its own peculiarities. One of the reasons you might have a weight problem is that you're an Indian. Our genetic make-up, diet and lifestyle push us towards obesity.

Globally, more than 1 billion people are overweight;[1] the WHO recently coined the term 'globesity' to describe the global epidemic of obesity. A quarter of affluent urban Indians are now obese, and obesity is increasing rapidly among urban schoolchildren. 'India's current National Family Health Survey indicates that more than 20 per cent of urban Indians are overweight or obese. In the north-western state of Punjab, nearly 40 per cent of all women are overweight or obese.'[2] With nearly 60 per cent of cardiac patients in the world being Indians, India tops the world charts in heart attack risk. It has been reported that about five people die per minute from coronary artery disease (CAD) in India. According to the WHO, deaths due to coronary heart disease (CHD) will double among Indians (in the time frame 1995–2025). What is even more

---

1 WHO Media Centre, 'Obesity and Overweight: Fact Sheet', uploaded May 2012, available online at http://www.who.int/mediacentre/factsheets/fs311/en/.

2 Goodhealthindia.in, 'Obesity: Silent Killer in India', available online at http://goodhealthindia.in/obesity.html.

disturbing is that the median age at which Indians tend to develop cardiovascular disease is 5–10 years lesser than in the rest of the world.

The International Diabetes Federation shows that every sixth diabetic in the world is an Indian—earning India the title of 'the world's diabetes capital'. Research over the past decade shows that genetically, Indians store more body fat per kilogram than Europeans. Leading health professionals agree that obesity puts Indians at an even greater risk of developing diabetes. Obesity in childhood is a major risk factor for future diabetes. According to the WHO, India will be the diabetic capital of the world by 2025 with 69.9 million people being diabetic. As with heart disease, a striking feature of diabetes among Indians is that the median age at which we develop it is 10–15 years lower than other populations, and the difference in diabetes rates is highest among those under 50.[3] The tendency to develop diabetes is seen among Indian children even in the absence of obesity.

---

3 R. Sicree, J. Shaw and P. Zimmet, 'Diabetes and Impaired Glucose Tolerance', *IDF Diabetes Journal* 3 (2006): 15–103.

Thrifty genes

All ancient populations were frequently subjected to selective pressure by famine, especially since the dawn of agriculture. The body adapts itself to these situations by lowering energy consumption. This is followed by a rapid deposition of energy as body fat in times of plenty to enable individuals to survive the periods of starvation. This is called the thrifty gene hypothesis.

Proponents of this theory use it to explain why certain populations, particularly Indians, or developing agricultural economies like India have a genetic predisposition to high levels of obesity and type 2 diabetes mellitus. Then there is the issue of our own genetics or family history. It is well known that obesity runs in families. Up to 40 per cent of the variation in body weight can be explained by genetic factors.

It is important, though, to recognize that the escalating epidemic of obesity in recent years cannot be explained by ethnic group susceptibility, as our gene pool is not known to change over thousands of years. Rather, rapid changes in environment and eating behaviour have contributed to this epidemic. What is clear, however, is that Indians are more susceptible to environmental and lifestyle changes compared to their Western counterparts. Further, family history or genes are not an excuse. Although you may have a genetic predisposition, obesity is more likely to be a result of the interaction between genes and environment, that is, even though you may be more prone to gaining weight, the solution lies in managing your environment. It just means that some of us may need to work harder to manage our weight.

The Indian diet

High-carbohydrate and high-glycaemic diets

While most traditional diets globally are centred on carbohydrates, particularly through cereals, Indian diets tend to have multiple staples—rice, wheat, potatoes, pulses—coupled with high levels of sweets and sugars through sweetened drinks and bakery. With the advent of modernization, cereals now undergo processing, which robs them of protective nutrients and fibre. A sharp increase in the consumption of refined carbohydrates since the 1960s has contributed to the epidemic of obesity in India.

On top of this, the high glycaemic index (GI) of Indian diets—a necessity for our ancestors' lifestyles—is not serving us well. GI ranks foods on the basis of their ability to raise blood sugar levels. Pure glucose has the highest GI—that is, 100—and raw, uncooked vegetables have among the lowest GI. High-GI foods are associated with obesity, metabolic syndrome, diabetes, dyslipidemia (abnormal cholesterol levels) and heart disease.

The myth of the Indian vegetarian diet

Vegetarians worldwide are far fitter, with normal lipid profiles and low rates of heart disease, than Indians. In a large-scale scientific study, nearly half the participants were lifelong vegetarians and yet the rates of obesity and heart disease were similar to those found among non-vegetarians. In fact, the rates of diabetes were actually higher among the vegetarians.[4] This is because the concept of vegetarianism is different among Indians, who eat large amounts of high-glycaemic carbohydrates, potatoes, fry food frequently and reuse the oil, and do not include enough raw foods, salads and fruits, which must be central to a good vegetarian diet.

Sugar and sweetened products

In India, our intake of sweets and sweetened drinks (sherbets, lemon water [nimbu-pani], etc.) is naturally very high. Additionally, our towns and cities are big consumers of aerated drinks.

Poor quality and nature of fats

Trans fats (also known as trans-fatty acids or TFAs), the most harmful kind of fat, have entered our diets in a big way through commercially available snacks, biscuits, cookies, fried foods and refined oils. The high intake of trans fats is associated with insulin resistance and weight gain around the abdomen. Indians, like most other Asians, have a tendency to accumulate girth around the abdomen, possibly due to diminished tolerance for trans fats.

Snacking

Snacking is a big part of the Indian diet. Traditional Indian snacks such as samosas, namkeens and bhujias are made out of highly refined

---

4 Enas A. Enas and Sudesh Kannan, 'Heart Disease in Particular Populations: Cracking the Indian Paradox' in *How to Beat the Heart Disease Epidemic among South Asians: A Prevention and Management Guide for Asian Indians and Their Doctors* (Illinois: Advanced Heart Lipid Clinic, 2005), 122.

and processed foods like refined flour (maida), polished rice, refined sugars, refined oils, etc., and many use oils with trans fats. We are also a nation of biscuit eaters. These foods, being easy to digest and low in satiety, make us feel hungry faster, thus increasing our risk of obesity. They are also low in protective nutrients like minerals, vitamins and antioxidants; this further increases our risk of developing metabolic abnormalities and obesity. While small, frequent meals with snacks are a good thing, the nature of those snacks makes all the difference.

Late dinners

While the world sits down for dinner in the evening after work, most urban Indians reach home to a snack with tea or drinks between 6 p.m. and 8 p.m. A 2007 survey by ACNielsen reported that the highest consumption of unhealthy snacks such as biscuits, chips and namkeens takes place pre-dinner. According to most diet recalls, people report peak hunger at this time. The consumption of unhealthy food and extra calories around this time ends up creating dietary disasters.

We also entertain in a very particular way—quite differently from how people entertain in the West. Socializing in India usually involves a few hours of drinking and unhealthy snacking, followed by a very late and heavy dinner. Eating high-carbohydrate and large meals late at night puts us at a hormonal disadvantage and favours easy fat deposition. Those who are insulin resistant are more vulnerable.

Indian hospitality

While food is the symbol of love and affection globally, in India it is even more so. The more you force a person to eat, the more warmth and affection you show. The traditional Indian *khaatir* or hospitality is so much a part of us that saying 'no' to food is often seen as rudeness.

There never seems to be a dull moment in the festival calendar either. There are approximately 140 festivals celebrated across the country in a year, perhaps the most any nation can boast of. Celebrations always include high-calorie, high-carbohydrate and high-fat sweets and savouries. Aloo-puri-halwa, kheer and the many mithais are the most typical north Indian foods of celebration. Then there are the several fasts, which are followed by feasts. Marriage itself is such an elaborate event, particularly in north India, with food as the central theme.

Staying still

Our domestic staff often outnumbers family members at home, and even in offices, there are plenty of clerks and peons to do the groundwork. A white-collar executive will have a chauffeur who not only drives him or her to the doorstep but also carries the laptop, lunch box and other baggage right into the cabin. Even schoolchildren from affluent families often follow the same routine. We rarely have to lift a finger if we don't want to.

A young mother, for example, will almost always have an exclusive maid and sometimes even a nurse to help her cope with her newborn baby. She may even be exempt from the burden of routine domestic chores—quite unlike the situation in the West. Alongside this, she is often advised to eat high-calorie foods like ghee, butter, cream, milk, nuts, etc. to regain her strength. No wonder most young mothers are found to be overweight in India.

Nor do we have a culture of walking or cycling through our cities, what with the broken footpaths and the hot weather. Mechanized means of transport, be it cars, elevators or escalators, have replaced walking, riding and biking almost completely. All these factors have radically reduced caloric requirements to a fraction of what they used to be as little as a generation ago.

This explains why India—a nation in transition—has become the world capital of diabetes and heart disease, and the rates of obesity are comparable to those found in the developed world.

Other general lifestyle factors that contribute to the epidemic of obesity

Increasing consumption of alcohol and junk or processed foods

Alcohol has empty calories and causes preferential deposition of fat, particularly around the abdomen. In fact, it may deplete the body of many precious nutrients, including vitamin B_1, zinc and magnesium, increasing your predisposition to obesity. Junk or processed foods are low in fibre and certain nutrients—calcium, magnesium, chromium and vitamin D—and have also been found to be associated with weight gain.

Supersizing, smart marketing and easy availability of unhealthy foods

Obesity is on the rise all over the First World but, as I have said earlier, in Indian cities and towns the levels of obesity are comparable to the levels in the developed world. The big reasons are the same—there is easy availability of cheap, unhealthy foods, our portion sizes have exploded (a cola in the 1970s was a little under 300 ml; today it can vary from 1–2 litres. A single order of popcorn was a cup and a half; today it is often a tub, which can be as much as 8–16 cups), and watching TV, playing video games and surfing the web have replaced outdoor activities for growing children. Those who watch 4 or more hours of TV are more likely to be overweight than those who watch less.[5] A multimillion-dollar advertising industry promotes appealing and enticing advertisements targeted at children and young adults to increase their desire to choose unhealthy foods. With economic affluence and the 24x7 availability of food, eating out has become more a way of life than just an indulgence, and the growing waistlines are not surprising.

Belly and the brain

While a lot has been said about genes, diet and other factors, a huge and largely undiscussed area is the relationship between our mind

5 J. Salmon and others, 'The Association between Television Viewing and Overweight among Australian Adults Participating in Varying Levels of Leisure-time Physical Activity', *International Journal of Obesity and Related Metabolic Disorders* 24, no. 5 (May 2000): 600–06.

and food. Many of us eat not to satisfy our hunger but to feed other needs. Emotions can drive us to eat for comfort or to cope with stress, boredom or happiness. Deep-rooted emotions, unresolved conflicts, unkind remarks and unpleasant experiences, even in early childhood, can alter your eating behaviour later in life, thus contributing to obesity. Abnormal eating behaviours such as binge eating, night eating, compulsive eating, food addiction, anorexia and bulimia have their origins in the mind.

In general, our relationship with food has undergone a change from a time when we used to eat to live to the present where, more often than not, we live to eat. The difference between hunger and appetite explains what drives us to eat more than what we need. Hunger defines the need to eat. Appeasing it creates satiety—that is, no further desire to eat exists. Appetite, in contrast, refers to the signals that guide dietary selection, often in the absence of obvious hunger. Appetite is usually associated with pleasure during food consumption and is mainly governed by external factors—religion, philosophy, cultural taboos, the presence of others, taste and palatability, preferences and aversions learnt by experience, anxiety, stress, psychological disturbances, environmental factors such as climate, metabolic factors (hormone levels, caloric requirements), aromas, mealtimes, memories and certain food advertisements—that influence our eating habits and patterns. We probably respond more to external, appetite-related forces than to hunger-related ones in choosing when and what to eat; this leads us to gain weight.

It also explains why a multidisciplinary approach is needed for the long-term success of weight management for many individuals.

Medical conditions and hormonal problems

Many people blame their hormones for their weight problems. True medical disorders that cause obesity are rare. Underactive thyroid (hypothyroidism) may cause weight gain because of a general slowing-down of metabolic activity; however, those treated with medication for it have little reason to blame the hormones.

Life-cycle phases associated with hormonal changes such as puberty, pregnancy, peri- and post-menopause or post-surgical menopause (hysterectomy) are high-risk times for weight gain. Leptin resistance and insulin resistance, secondary to poor diet and lifestyle choices, can predispose you to weight gain. Leptin is a hormone that plays an important role in appetite regulation, suppressing food intake and inducing weight loss. Long-term consumption of refined and processed foods that are high in sugar and fat content induces leptin resistance, which is a hallmark of obesity.

Other medical problems associated with weight gain include:

Down's syndrome

Reduced metabolic rate combined with Down's syndrome may cause weight gain.

Cushing's syndrome

In contrast to adults, children with Cushing's syndrome may have generalized obesity accompanied by slow linear growth.

Growth Hormone Deficiency (GHD)

The gradual decline in growth hormone with age may in part explain the increase in visceral or abdominal fat.

Medications

Certain drugs and treatments that are associated with weight gain include chemotherapy during cancer treatment, steroid hormones, hormone therapy particularly for polycystic ovarian syndrome, in vitro fertilization (IVF), contraception, tricyclic antidepressants, anticonvulsants, anti-diabetic agents, insulin and some anti-hypertensives.

Some general factors that lead to weight gain

Ageing

As you age, the amount of muscle in your body tends to decrease, thus lowering metabolic rate and increasing the risk of obesity.

Gender

Obesity affects both men and women, with some notable gender-specific differences. More men than women are in the overweight category, but more women than men are in the obese category.

Occupation

People in professions that require them to be around food—chefs, bakers, tasters, caterers, food critics, hotel, restaurant and sweet shop owners—have been known to be associated with higher rates of obesity compared to others.

Very active professionals like dancers and sportspeople also tend to become victims of obesity as they move out of active professional life. Night-shift and BPO workers too are prone to weight gain, owing to disrupted circadian rhythms and poor lifestyles.

Stopping smoking

Smokers tend to gain some weight after giving up smoking, usually up to 2–5 kg. About one out of ten ex-smokers gain as much as 12–15 kg, after they quit smoking—with more weight being gained in the first 6 months.

Post-illness or bed rest

Bed rest and prolonged illness may also lead to excess weight. Often, genetically predisposed children recovering from illnesses like hepatitis or typhoid can gain large amounts of weight, which may persist due to the intake of high-carbohydrate diets, sweetened juices, etc. People on wheelchairs, or with medical conditions such as arthritis, joint and knee pains, fractures, etc. that limit activity, often experience weight gain.

Chronic dieting, fad diets and information overload

Chronic/frequent dieters find it hard or are unable to lose weight and maintain it. The reason behind this is that each time we lose weight, our metabolic rate drops and the body slows down and hoards calories, making it harder for us to lose weight the next time around.

Fad diets constitute a short-term, quick-fix approach to weight loss and do not work over the long haul. These diets tend to over-promise results but fail to deliver. The food choices they offer are monotonous and the caloric intake restricted, which ends up wearing off the motivation to continue. Such faddy regimens neither encourage healthy eating nor establish safe and permanent weight loss.

An overload of confusing, conflicting and contradicting details about food and theories of weight management often result in failure. Disillusioned by diets, many get demotivated and give up.

Sleep

Individuals who don't get sufficient sleep or experience sleep disorders like chronic insomnia and sleep apnoea have been found to be at an increased risk of obesity.

Friends and family

Having unfit people around can make you feel comfortable and complacent; also, your benchmark for size stretches to being more liberal than stringent. Unhealthy friends also tend to encourage you to eat like them.

Exam time

The burden of exams, especially in our country, brings with it unending tuitions and prolonged stress accompanied by high-calorie snacking. To make matters worse, exercise and sports come to a grinding halt. Stress eating and parental indulgence too add up, leading to the piling up of calories. Consequently, this has been found to be a time when most students end up putting on extra kilos—anything from 2–15 kg—in a span of few months.

Studying or living away from home

Often children and adolescents studying away from home, or people living away from family, are seen to be at risk of overweight and obesity.

Holidaying and frequent travelling

These can change fitness routines and food choices, making you prone to gaining weight.

✚ ADDING IT ALL UP

In Chapter 1 you learnt how to calculate how much weight you need to lose. Now I have also talked about the key factors that may lead to weight gain. This chapter really forms the bedrock of the book. I hope it has also helped you understand why you might be overweight or find it difficult to shed the weight. The Indian context—our genetic make-up, environment and lifestyle—is a very peculiar one. Hence, Indians might need to put in greater efforts to manage their weight, and diets need to be customized as per individual needs.

[illegible] of calories. Consequently, this [illegible] to the time when most students end up putting on extra kilos – anything from a [illegible] kg in a span of few months.

Studying or living away from home

Often children and adolescents studying away from home (or people living away from family) are seen to be at risk of overweight and obesity.

Holidaying and frequent travelling

These can change fitness routines and food choices, making you prone to gaining weight.

✚ ADDING IT ALL UP

[illegible] [illegible]

3

CALORIES AND NUTRIENTS: THE BUILDING BLOCKS

✚ THE DOCTOR SAYS

The only way you can lose weight, enjoy feeling lighter and stay fit is if you mind what you eat, constantly and consistently. Knowledge of calories and nutrients is a great tool to manage your everyday diet. Though I don't want you to count calories all the time, a broad understanding and a general sense of how nutrients help and how much of them you need to have will help you manage your weight better. Some basic principles of healthy eating along with this will help you understand why I am suggesting what I am. I think it always helps to do something with understanding rather than to follow things blindly. I have observed that the more aware my clients are, the more likely they are to stick to their meal plans.

Understanding calories

All foods provide energy. Energy is commonly expressed in kilocalories (kcal) or kilojoules (kJ). The use of the term 'calorie' with regard to food is, strictly speaking, inaccurate. A calorie is actually an energy unit used in physics and chemistry, defined as the energy needed to heat a gram of water by 1°C. In contrast, the calorie that we talk about with regard to food measures how much energy we derive from food. A dietary calorie is actually 1000 calories. That is why you mostly see the abbreviation 'kcal' on the nutrition panels on the labels of products.

A very important tool in weight management is to understand how many calories your diet provides. If your diet provides more calories than you need you are in positive calorie balance, which leads to weight gain, overweight and obesity. If your diet provides the same number of calories as your body requires, you are able to maintain your weight.

While being calorie-wise is good, according to my clinical experience, too much emphasis on calories is not warranted and may be counterproductive. In fact, what those calories are made up of is more important, that is, the break-up of different nutrients—carbohydrates, proteins and fats—is equally important, if not more. This means that even if you are on a low-calorie diet (say, 1000 kcal), if all these calories come only from carbohydrates amounting to 250 gm—which is equivalent to 50 tsp of sugar, which in turn is equal to six cans of sweetened cola—weight loss is unlikely. No wonder the typical 1000 kcal diets, consisting of six cereals (chapattis) along with a serving of vegetables, dal, yogurt (dahi), a fruit and a couple of biscuits in a day, may not result in weight loss for many as they are high in carbohydrates with inadequate proteins and nutrients.

Calories come from three chief nutrients:

1. Carbohydrates : 4 kcal/gm
2. Proteins : 4 kcal/gm
3. Fats : 9 kcal/gm

Individual caloric requirements

An individual's caloric requirements are determined by:

Basal Metabolic Rate (BMR)

BMR determines 60–65 per cent of the total caloric requirement. Such calories are required by the body for metabolism at rest. A heavy individual has a higher BMR than a lean person.

Physical activity

Physical activity determines 25–30 per cent of the total caloric requirement. Such calories are required to perform daily physical work.

Thermic effect of food

The thermic effect of food determines 10 per cent of the total caloric requirement. Such calories are associated with the metabolism of food, that is, digestion, absorption and storage of energy. The thermic effect of proteins is higher than that of fats and carbohydrates.

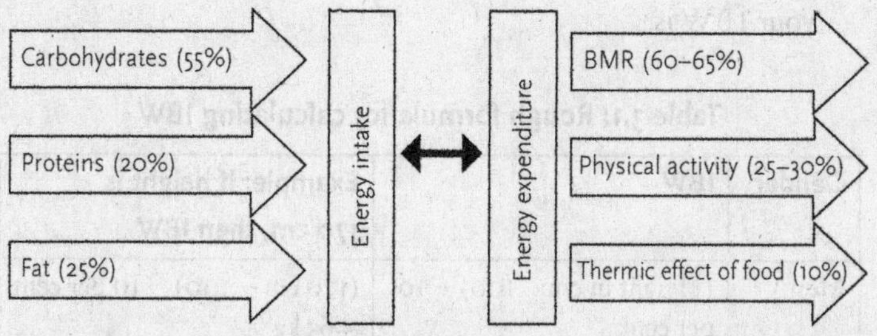

Clearly, the more energy we expend, the more efficiently we lose weight. We all vary considerably in our basal metabolic rates; this is one of the key reasons why individual caloric requirements need to be calculated and customized. We can increase our BMR by improving our lean body mass or muscle mass. Therefore, resistance and weight-bearing exercises, which help increase muscle mass and in turn increase our BMR, are important. We can increase the number of calories burnt through physical activity by movement, also called NEAT (non-exercise-associated thermogenesis), and engaging in physical activity and sports.

We can increase the thermic effect of food by having more raw vegetables and adequate protein. **Lowering the intake of calories through the right diet along with increasing the expenditure of energy through physical activity is the right way to lose weight.**

How to calculate your caloric requirements

How many calories you require depends upon your body weight and physical activity.

1. Know your ideal body weight: A rough formula for calculating your IBW is:

Table 3.1: Rough formula for calculating IBW

Gender	IBW	Example: If height is 170 cm, then IBW
Men	(Height in cm – 100) – 10 per cent	(170 cm – 100) – 10 per cent = 63 kg
Women	(Height in cm – 100) – 15 per cent	(170 cm – 100) – 15 per cent = 60 kg

2. Based on your IBW, calculate your caloric requirements.

Table 3.2: Method to calculate individual calorie requiremnts

Individual cases	**Caloric requirements**	**Example: If IBW is 60 kg**
To achieve IBW	25 kcal/kg × IBW	1500 kcal
For those who engage in moderate activity*	30 kcal/kg × IBW	1800 kcal
For the overweight	15–20 kcal/kg × IBW	900–1200 kcal
For the underweight	30 kcal/kg × IBW	1800 kcal
For the underweight who engage in moderate activity	35 kcal/kg × IBW	2100 kcal
For endurance athletes	50–80 kcal/kg × IBW	3000–4800 kcal

* Moderate activity refers to everyday activities which require some physical strain such as doing housework, brisk walking, active interaction and playing with children, gardening, etc.

Individual requirements can vary hugely, amounting to a difference of almost 1000 kcal per day per person. Usually, 20–30 kcal per kg of IBW is adequate to maintain your IBW. A deficit of 500 kcal per day will help you lose half a kilogram of fat in a week.

It has been found that 1 gm of body fat (adipose tissue) provides 7 kcal and to lose ½ kg fat, we need to burn 3500 kcal, which requires a deficit of 500 kcal a day. Simply put, 500 kcal x 7 days = 3500 kcal = ½ kg loss of body fat in a week.

For safe and long-term weight loss, you are recommended to lose ½–1 kg of weight a week, which averages to about 2–4 kg a month. Variations exist as individuals lose more or less; the average over months still works out to be about the same. Quick weight loss is highly undesirable as it forces the body to use proteins (muscles) instead of fat for energy and lowers your BMR.

Weight-loss diets usually range from an average of 800–1200 kcal per day, while very low calorie diets (VLCDs) can go down to as low as 600 kcal per day. Such low-calorie diets are safe only under supervision and for short spells of time, no more than a few weeks or months.

Understanding nutrients

Carbohydrates

These are the critical nutrients affecting body weight and have caused much debate in the area of weight management. Both the quantity and quality of carbohydrates are hugely important for weight loss, particularly for individuals with insulin resistance. Several studies have reported the benefits of lowering carbohydrate calories and stepping up protein and fat. People with metabolic obesity, diabetes or a positive family history of diabetes, and women with conditions associated with hormonal imbalance (such as PCOS) experience better results by lowering their carbohydrate intake.

Sugars, sweets, fruits and grains/cereals are the chief sources of carbohydrates. Legumes, dairy and vegetables also provide carbohydrates. The quantity of carbohydrates, that is, the percentage of calories obtained from carbohydrates, is crucial. Traditional diets provide for up to 60–70 per cent of the total caloric requirement through carbohydrates. But most of us can do with cutting down our carbohydrate intake to 45–50 per cent of our diet.

For effective weight loss, remember the following:

1. Distribute carbohydrates over the course of the day—don't load up on carbohydrates in one meal or late at night.
2. Fifteen–thirty gm of carbohydrates in six small meals might be helpful.
3. Small, frequent meals rev up metabolism and promote weight loss.

Table 3.3: Serving sizes of foods for 15 gm of carbohydrate

Food type	Serving sizes
Fruits	1 cup high–water content fruits (melon and berries) ½ cup most fruits ½ banana ¼ cup dry fruits ⅛ cup dry/sweet fruits (raisins or dried banana chips)
Grains, pulses and starchy vegetables	3 cups popcorn 1 cup puffed cereals 1 slice bread ½ cup pasta (cooked)/dry vegetables (potato)/ sweet vegetables (corn, peas, winter squash) ½ cup pulses/dals/beans ⅓ cup rice ¼ cup dry/sweet vegetables (yam [jimikand] or sweet potato)

Food type	Serving sizes
Low-carbohydrate vegetables*	3 cups raw vegetables (high in water/low in sweetness) 1½ cups vegetables (cooked); (high in water/low in sweetness
Milk	1 cup milk or yogurt (unsweetened)

* Do not count low-carbohydrate vegetables under 'carbohydrates' unless they provide about 15 gm or more of carbohydrates.

Concentrated carbohydrate sources

1 tsp sugar = 4 gm carbohydrates
½ cup sugar = 95 gm carbohydrates
1 tbsp flour = 5 gm carbohydrates
½ cup flour = 45 gm carbohydrates

Types of carbohydrates

Besides the quantity, the type or quality of carbohydrates also has an impact on weight loss. Carbohydrates are classified on the basis of their glycaemic indices. Glucose is given a reference of 100 and other foods are rated accordingly. They are categorized as:

Low–glycaemic index carbohydrates (<50)

These are good and 'slow' carbohydrates. The slower the carbohydrates, the steadier the supply of energy you get from their intake and the more full and energized you feel. Low–glycaemic index foods are recommended for most urban sedentary individuals, for weight loss and for diabetics. They are high in fibre and other essential nutrients—vitamins, minerals and antioxidants. Whole grains such as oats, barley, quinoa, lentils, beans, nuts, seeds, raw and cooked vegetables and most fruits are low–glycaemic index foods.

High–glycaemic index carbohydrates (>50)

These carbohydrates are easily digested and absorbed, thereby raising blood sugar levels rapidly. High–glycaemic index foods are needed to keep energy levels high during sports, physical activity or recovery from illness. This induces a surge of insulin response which rapidly brings down sugars, making you crave for more. High–glycaemic index foods are best eaten in combination with protein- and fat-rich foods, or low–glycaemic index foods. Sugars, polished rice, wheat, refined wheat flour, semolina (sooji), noodles, idli, dosa, naan, cornflakes, corn, fruit juices and potatoes are some examples of high–glycaemic index carbohydrates.

Take home

1. Low–glycaemic index diets are far more suitable for weight loss.
2. Limit intake of sugar and sweets. Count these under 'total carbohydrates' in a meal. (One tsp of sugar amounts to 4 gm of carbohydrates.)
3. Very low–carbohydrate diets (with less than 100 gm of carbohydrates) are lower in vitamins, minerals and phytochemicals (disease-fighting chemicals) and may put you at risk of heart disease, osteoporosis, arthritis and digestive problems.
4. Excessive intake of carbohydrates causes weight gain and obesity, and increases the risk of developing high triglycerides those with metabolic syndrome and central obesity (see section on the apple shape, p. 12).

Proteins

These are essential for the growth and repair of tissues. Rich sources include meat, eggs, low-fat dairy, legumes and nuts. Grains/cereals and vegetables have very little protein. Animal proteins from eggs, milk, fish and poultry are complete proteins, which means they contain all the essential amino acids (building blocks of proteins) needed by the body. Plant proteins from grains/cereals and pulses are incomplete proteins individually, but a combination of grains/cereals and pulses makes for complete proteins.

Fifteen–twenty per cent of your total calories should come from proteins. Alternatively, 0.75–1 gm of protein per kg of IBW is the recommended daily allowance. About 60 gm of protein per day is more than enough for most people. Women may need about 40–50 gm per day, while men may require 55–60 gm per day.

Excess protein intake can tilt the pH balance of the body, which can lead to hyperacidity, digestive complaints, muscle pains and strained kidneys, and may eventually lead to kidney damage. It may also increase cholesterol levels, risk of heart disease, and the levels of uric acid in the blood, which may lead to joint pains and gout. Animal protein especially, if taken in excess, could leach calcium from bones which may increase the risk of osteoporosis.

Low-protein diets may be low on satiety, promote water retention, increase inflammation and cravings, and, over a long period, can promote weight gain. They may cause muscle soreness, and loss in lean body mass, especially for those engaging in physical exercise and weight training. Remember, inadequate protein intake too can interfere with weight loss.

Do protein shakes play a significant role during weight loss?

Well-planned diets will be able to meet protein needs through normal food for most people. Protein shakes or supplements limit variety and do not provide all the benefits of food (like phytochemicals) or a sense of satisfaction. Remember, excess proteins can also lead to weight gain. These supplements do not enable you to choose food proactively, thereby making it difficult to sustain long-term weight loss.

How much protein to eat

1. Aim for 4–6 servings per day of protein-rich foods on most days. (See Table 3.4 for serving sizes.)
2. Try to consume at least 1–2 servings per day of low-fat milk, yogurt or soy milk.
3. A combination of one or more protein-rich foods—pulses, lentils, nuts, seeds, lean meats, chicken, fish and eggs—must be a part of your diet.
4. A generous serving of vegetables will provide plant proteins.

Table 3.4: Protein content of commonly consumed foods

Food type	Serving sizes	Protein (gm)
Cheese	⅛ cup	7
Cottage cheese (paneer)	¼ cup	7
Dal (boiled and drained) or boiled beans	½ cup	7
Egg	1 (50 gm)	7

Food type	Serving sizes	Protein (gm)
Grain/cereals	1 chapatti/½ cup rice or pasta or noodle (cooked)	2–3
Lean meat, fish and poultry	100 gm	20–24
Milk	1 cup	8
Nuts	¼ cup	7
Tofu	½ cup	7
Vegetables (cut up)	½ cup	2
Yogurt	1 cup	8

Fats

These are a concentrated source of energy and provide satiety. They are essential for absorption of fat-soluble vitamins—A, D, E and K. Nuts, seeds, meat, eggs, fatty fish, low-fat dairy and cooking oils are key sources of fat in our diet.

About 20–30 per cent of your total caloric intake must come from fats. Don't believe me? Research shows that a 30 per cent fat content seems to offer more benefits, particularly for those who suffer from excessive hunger or cravings. This is because foods with good-quality fats and good-quality protein along with adequate fibre appear to diminish hunger and control cravings. Nuts, seeds, whole grains, legumes, sprouts, soy, fruit and vegetable salads with legumes, low-fat dairy, yogurt, fruits and cheese may be helpful.

Very low fat diets do not provide satiety. They are usually inherently high in carbohydrates, making insulin-resistant or metabolically obese individuals more vulnerable to heart disease. They may lead to rapid weight loss, which could be damaging as it may lead to excessive loss of muscle, and essential fatty acid deficiency (resulting in hair fall and endocrine problems), and increase the risk of developing gallstones.

Types of fats

Depending on their biochemical composition, fats are classified into three types. An optimum balance of all three is needed for good health.

Saturated fatty acids (SFAs)

Foods with SFAs are solid at room temperature. Butter, ghee and coconut are good sources of these fats. Saturated fats in excess can lead to increased levels of bad cholesterol (LDL) and triglycerides (blood fats).

Monounsaturated fatty acids (MUFAs)

Foods with MUFAs are liquid at room temperature. They lower bad cholesterol (LDL), improve good cholesterol (HDL) and also help prevent gallstones. MUFA-rich oils help in improving insulin metabolism and thereby help in reducing belly fat. Good sources of MUFAs include olive, canola, mustard, sesame and groundnut oils.

Polyunsaturated fatty acids (PUFAs)

Foods with PUFAs are also liquid at room temperature. They lower both bad cholesterol (LDL) and good cholesterol (HDL). Polyunsaturated fats can be obtained from oils such as sunflower, safflower, corn and soybean. They also provide essential fats—

omega-3 and omega-6 fatty acids. An optimum balance between omega-3 and omega-6 fats is needed for good health as an excess of omega-6 fats can cause health problems.

Omega-3 fats are known to have anti-inflammatory properties, boost metabolism, and enhance immunity and fat burning. They are in fact wonder fats with a great number of health benefits. Fish oils and fatty fishes (hilsa, katla, surmai, black pomfret and salmon), seeds (flax, chia, mustard, sesame and fenugreek), rice bran oil, green leafy vegetables, bajra, soybeans, rajma, black gram (urad dal) and black-eyed beans (lobiya) are good sources of omega-3 fats.

However, excessive amounts (>7 per cent of total calories) of PUFA-rich oils can interfere with insulin metabolism, compromise immunity, increase inflammation and promote the formation of gallstones.

Other fats

Conjugated linoleic acids (CLAs)

These are a type of fat found in dairy products including milk. They have been found to reduce fat deposition, possibly through increased fat oxidation and decreased triglyceride uptake in adipose (fat) tissue. However, currently there is no human data to support the theory that CLAs are effective during weight loss.

Medium-chain triglycerides (MCTs)

These are found in coconut and virgin coconut oil, and have been found to have special health benefits particularly during weight loss. They appear to help by controlling food intake and energy expenditure. It is believed that energy expenditure is also greater following the consumption of a meal with MCTs. During a 12-week study people lost significantly more body fat consuming MCTs on a daily basis.[1] Insulin response with MCTs is also lower. It must be noted that MCTs are really only effective when they replace other fats, not when they are added to your original fat intake.

✚ ADDING IT ALL UP

Calories are the building blocks of our food—and the key to weight loss. But it's not that simple. The aim is to lessen our total intake of calories, while choosing the right quality of calories. This chapter should have given you a greater understanding of the three key nutrients. However, most of the foods we eat contain a combination of these nutrients. And so to make it easier for my clients, I break up the food that they eat on the basis of food groups rather than nutrients. More on this in the next chapter.

1 M.L. Assunção and others, 'Effects of Dietary Coconut Oil on the Biochemical and Anthropometric Profiles of Women Presenting Abdominal Obesity', *Lipids* 44, no. 2 (July 2009): 593–601.

4

FOOD GROUPS AND PORTION CONTROL

✚ THE DOCTOR SAYS

Now that you are familiar with nutrients, you must understand that nature provides all these nutrients to us through a variety of foods. Some foods have more, some less and most contain combinations; they have been grouped into food groups accordingly. For example, cereals and fruits are predominantly carbohydrates, meats and eggs are predominantly proteins, nuts are combinations of fats and proteins, and milk is a combination of proteins, fats and carbohydrates.

As you absorb the idea of food groups, you will begin to look at the food on your plate differently and classify it according to the group it most fits into. For example, a salad with walnuts falls under the 'vegetable' group. If two groups figure equally in the composition of a food, it may fall under both groups. So palak paneer may fall under both 'vegetable' and 'dairy'. The ability to classify food in this manner will not only help you identify the right foods for your body but it will also help you make wise food choices throughout your life. **Knowing food groups and practising portion control are the two fundamentals of my diet.**

Grains/cereals

These constitute the foundation of most diets in the world and provide carbohydrates, the chief fuel for the body. Staples tend to give a characteristic identity to cuisines and cultures, becoming almost symbolic of the region in question—for example, take the case of chapatti (north India), rice (south and east India), dosa (south India), breads (Europe and North America), pasta (Italy), and noodles and rice (Asia). Traditionally, staples sit at the base of the food pyramid and represent the largest area.

While this group was certainly critical to ancient societies where manual work was the norm, the relevance of this group in our current society has changed. With energy requirements and caloric needs falling drastically, the requirements of this group have dropped too. Grain/cereal requirements must be appropriate to the level of energy expended in physical activity and fulfilling the needs of the body. **This means that most of our energy requirements need no longer be obtained from this group alone. However, at least half the day's cereal intake must be provided through whole grains.**

Grain-/cereal-free diets are nutritionally fine and, if planned well, can even help to reverse insulin resistance. The Palaeolithic diet, for example, consists mainly of lean meat, fish, vegetables, fruits, roots, tubers and nuts. Remember that cutting down on grains/cereals doesn't mean that you are cutting down on carbohydrates as they are also available through other sources like fruits, pulses, milk, curd and vegetables.

Adequate grains/cereals, however, reduce the risk of obesity, CAD, diabetes, cancer and several other chronic diseases. It also keeps the digestive system healthy, provides bulk and promotes fullness as well as the growth of friendly bacteria (probiotics), which have been linked to profound health benefits.

Including the right type of grains/cereals based on their glycaemic index has a huge impact on weight control and reduction of belly fat. Choosing low–glycaemic index cereals, like barley, soy, pulses, oats and quinoa, helps increase fullness, lower cravings, improve energy and concentration, improve hormone regulation, correct irregular menstruation, and control acne, dandruff and facial hair growth. Besides weight control they are also useful in reducing blood glucose and cholesterol levels, thereby being useful in controlling diabetes and heart disease.

Nutrients

Grains/cereals provide complex carbohydrates, fibre, vitamins B_1, B_3, B_6 and E, folic acid, iron, selenium, zinc and antioxidants.

Servings per day

One serving of grains/cereals provides 70–80 kcal roughly. On an average, 5–8 servings of grains/cereals a day are appropriate for a moderately active person. However, for those trying to lose weight, portion size may be reduced to as little as 2–4 servings a day.

Table 4.1: Serving sizes of commonly consumed grains/cereals

Grains/cereals	1 serving
Bread	1 (medium) slice
Bagel	¼ (large)
Bhatura	½
Biscuits	2–3
Boiled corn	½ cup
Bread roll	1 (medium)

Grains/cereals	**1 serving**
Corn on the cob (bhutta)	½ (medium)
Chapatti	1 (medium)
Crackers	6
Dry flour	3 tbsp
French fries	1 cup/10 pcs
Hamburger/hot dog bun	½ bun
Idli	1 (large)
Kulcha	1
Muesli/granola	¼ cup/3 tbsp
Naan (8"x2")	⅓
Noodles (cooked)	½ cup
Pasta (cooked)	½ cup
Pita bread	½ (medium)
Pizza (thin crust)	2 (medium) slices
Plain dosa	1 (medium)/length of a table knife
Poha/upma (cooked)	½ cup
Popcorn	3 cups
Porridge (cooked)	½ cup
Potato*	1 (medium)
Potato chips	⅓ cup
Puffed cereal like puffed rice (murmura)	1½ cups
Rice (cooked)	½ cup
Roasted rice flakes (chirwa)	⅓ cup/3–4 tbsp
Sandwich	1 triangle/rectangle

* In nutrition science, potatoes and starchy vegetables like colocasia (arbi), sweet potatoes and yam are not a part of the 'fruit' or 'vegetable' groups and are included under 'grains/cereals', owing to their high carbohydrate content.

Whole versus refined grains

Increasingly, modern diets have shifted from whole grains to refined ones. With the epidemic of obesity, diabetes and other lifestyle diseases, the benefits of whole grains are being rediscovered. Traditional grains like whole wheat, millets, oats, barley and brown rice, lost in the fast-food jungle, are regaining popularity.

What is it that distinguishes whole grains from refined ones? Refining of cereal grains is historical and the debate over this subject has been found in biblical records. As refined grains were associated with social status and the wealthy could afford them, most preferred white flour and white rice over brown, even at the price of lost nutrients. Hippocrates, the father of modern medicine, however, advised his wealthy patrons to follow the practice of servants and to shift to whole grains to cure diseases.

Before the roller-mill revolution, wheat was ground between big stone wheels, which removed the bran from the wheat kernel and left the germ intact. The germ, high in nutrients (proteins and B vitamins including folic acid and oils), merely got crushed and released the oil; this shortened its life as the oil got rancid. This was overcome by the advent of rollers around the Industrial Revolution which made it possible to remove the germ and the bran and provided the pure white flour that produced light and fluffy bakery, which could be stored for months. This white flour became one of the staples of Western diets and a product of modern industrialized foods. The same was true of corn (cornflakes) and white rice. Wherever these refining technologies came into widespread use (particularly in the poorer regions), the epidemics of pellagra (deficiency of vitamin B_3) and beriberi (deficiency of vitamin B_1) came about due to the loss of

B vitamins present in the germ, lost during refining.

Refining grains extends their shelf life. It also makes them easier to digest by removing the fibre that normally slows down the release of carbohydrates. Also, the finer a grain is ground, the greater is the resultant flour's surface area exposed to digestive enzymes, and the quicker is its digestion. In other words, the starches convert into glucose. This phenomenon contributes to weight gain and obesity.

Research has established that a diet rich in whole grains has several health benefits including reduced risk of coronary artery disease, cancer, diabetes, obesity and several chronic diseases.[1] Due to their slow digestibility, whole grains/cereals help maintain blood sugar levels. **Whole grains, being high in fibre and low in fat, are also a good choice for weight-watchers.**

No one nutrient alone can be credited for the benefits of whole-grain foods. A whole food might be more than the sum of its nutrient parts. The special disease-protecting benefits come from numerous non-nutrient components. Among these are lignans, tocotrienols, phenolic compounds, phytic acid, tannins and enzyme inhibitors. These too are lost during the refining process!

The fibre in whole grains, besides keeping the digestive system healthy, providing bulk and helping in cholesterol reduction, also has a prebiotic effect as it promotes growth of friendly bacteria. Friendly bacteria or probiotics currently constitute a huge area of research as they are believed to have a far-reaching impact on health.

---

1 S.S. Jonnalagadda and others, 'Putting the Whole Grain Puzzle Together: Health Benefits Associated with Whole Grains—Summary of American Society for Nutrition 2010 Satellite Symposium', *The Journal of Nutrition* 141, no. 5 (May 2011): 1011S–22S.

Whole grains contain no cholesterol, are low in fat, high in dietary fibre and complex carbohydrates, and provide plant proteins, essential fatty acids, vitamins and minerals. They provide key vitamins and minerals like vitamin E (a powerful antioxidant), iron (needed for haemoglobin formation), selenium, zinc and B vitamins, including vitamin B_6 and folic acid. Vitamins E and B_6, folic acid, zinc and selenium are also powerful antioxidants that help in preventing several diseases including heart disease.

Current dietary recommendations in India, based on the food pyramid, support an increased consumption of whole grains, which should comprise at least half of the cereals we consume. In addition, a part of the recommended Indian health policy issued by the WHO is to ensure the production and availability of whole-grain cereals such as wheat and partially polished rice.

Choosing whole grains and whole grain–based products, like brown rice, whole-wheat breads, whole-grain breakfast cereals like muesli/granola and whole-wheat pastas and pizzas, instead of those made from refined flour or polished rice, can help combat the rising epidemic of chronic degenerative disorders. It is time to turn the wheel around and rediscover your roots.

> Myth: Combining two carbohydrates is not advisable—rice and chapatti together, for example, can cause weight gain.
>
> Fact: Variety is the spice of life. Combining two carbohydrates is not the issue; it is the quality and quantity of the carbohydrates that are important. You can happily consume 1 chapatti and ½ cup rice instead of 2 chapattis.

Myth: Semolina is a whole grain.
Fact: Semolina is a high-glycaemic refined grain. It is a granular form of refined flour. Its nutritional content is the same as any other refined grain like polished rice or refined wheat flour.

Myth: Brown bread is always healthy.
Fact: In India brown bread is very often coloured with caramel colour and may have only a small percentage of whole-wheat flour (atta). To be genuinely labelled 'whole wheat', it must be at least 50 per cent whole wheat.

Myth: Rice is more fattening than wheat.
Fact: Rice and wheat have the same percentage of carbohydrates. What matters is the amount you consume. Half a cup rice (cooked) = 1 (medium) chapatti. However, chapatti, brown rice and low-glycaemic rice have a higher satiety value than polished rice. Therefore you need more polished rice to feel full which leads to extra carbohydrates and calories, causing weight gain.

Myth: Potatoes, bread, pasta and rice are fattening.
Fact: Potatoes, bread, pasta and rice are starches high in carbohydrates, but not all carbohydrates are equal in terms of their effect on the body. Know your grain/cereal servings and manage accordingly. Count potatoes under your grain/cereal allowance.

Pulses

'Pulses', as a food group, includes all dals, lentils, peas, beans (rajma, black-eyed beans, soybean), gram, chickpeas, gram flour, sambar, sprouts, roasted gram (bhuna chana), pulse-based preparations (such as vadas, cheelas, vadis, dokhlas), textured soy protein (granules and chunks), etc. With a low glycaemic index, this group is extremely valuable for obesity management and controlling insulin resistance, especially for those with metabolic obesity, belly fat, PCOS or diabetes. Pulses are an excellent substitute for grains/cereals in the Indian context.

Nutrients

Nutrients are rich sources of proteins, fibre, desirable carbohydrates, B vitamins and zinc. They are a good source of plant protein, particularly for vegetarians. They are low in fat and free of cholesterol. Sprouted pulses contain additional vitamin C, an increased amount of B vitamins and valuable enzymes which cooked pulses do not have. Sprouts are exceptionally useful for weight management as they are extremely filling.

Servings per day

One serving of pulses provides roughly 70–80 kcal. Include at least 2–3 servings of pulses a day, if you are a vegetarian, but if you're on a weight-management regimen, 1–2 servings may be adequate. For non-vegetarians, pulse portions may need to be adjusted according to their intake of animal proteins: the total pulse intake should be between 1 and 2 servings. An excessive amount of this food group in your diet can lead to flatulence, bloating, and digestive disorders, particularly for those who are sensitive to them.

Table 4.2: Serving sizes of commonly consumed pulses

Pulse	1 serving
Beans (cooked)	½ cup
Cheela	2 (medium)/1 compact disc
Gram (roasted)	3 tbsp
Hummus	⅓ cup
Pulse (cooked)	1 cup
Pulse/chikpea/gram flour (besan)	3 tbsp

Soy

For vegetarians, soybean is a very good source of protein. Compared to other pulses and legumes, soy has almost double the amount of protein. Just about 1 serving (30 gm) of soybean provides an amount of protein almost similar to that obtained from non-vegetarian food items.

Sprouts

Sprouts are little food factories because they can create vitamins and enzymes within themselves. The enzymes help with digestion as they help break down proteins, fats and carbohydrates. One serving of sprouts is enough to meet an average adult's recommended daily need of 40 mg of vitamin C. Sprouts increase the levels of B vitamin in the body phenomenally, almost by 20–30 per cent, particularly with regard to vitamin B_1, folic acid and biotin.

Almost any whole bean, pulse, seed or grain can be sprouted. The most common sprouts remain moong bean, black gram (kala chana), chickpeas (safed chana), alfalfa, sunflower seeds and fenugreek (methi). However, soybean, sesame seeds (til) and millets are also good for sprouting. Alfalfa sprouts have special benefits as they contain compounds called saponins. Saponins have been found to lower bad cholesterol and stimulate the immune system.

> Myth: Rajma, chana and dals lead to weight gain.
> Fact: Rajma, chana and dals, just like soybean, are a wonderful source of plant protein. They also provide soluble fibre and good carbohydrates, and have a low glycaemic index. Remember, an excess of these can make you gassy.

> Myth: Cereals and pulses should not be eaten together.
> Fact: Food combinations seem to be bothering many. There is absolutely no basis for such beliefs. Foods naturally come in combinations of carbohydrates and proteins; for example, cereals and pulses are a combination of carbohydrates and proteins. In fact, combinations make for complete proteins.

Vegetables

Vegetables constitute the foundation for weight management and weight loss. They constitute a low-calorie, nutrient-dense food group, high in water content, fibre, micronutrients and antioxidants, and minerals like magnesium and potassium. They are aptly called functional foods. **Make sure you include all vegetables available at the local vendor. Do note that cottage cheese, beans (rajma, black-eyed beans), gram and potatoes do not belong to this group, as many vegetarians like to believe.**

Raw vegetables and some fruits are often referred to as 'negative calories', as they supposedly take more energy to process and digest than they provide (see section on wonder foods, p. 67). Several studies have shown that people consuming diets rich in vegetables have been able to lose weight and keep it off for longer. Diets rich in vegetables also reduce the risk of several diseases. Green leafy vegetables are a rich source of omega-3 fats (present in fish), the kind of fats that are helpful in weight management and provide protection from inflammatory conditions like heart disease, arthritis and asthma.

Vegetables are your single biggest allies on your path to weight loss. A cup of raw vegetables provides anything between 25 and 30 kcal, while a slice of cake or a brownie could be as much as 250 kcal. This means that you could eat 10–12 cups of raw vegetables and get as many calories as you would get from a slice of cake or a brownie. While the cake/brownie may provide very little nutrition and get you hungry within a short period of time, the vegetables will fulfil recommended daily allowances of several nutrients, and will help fill you up and feel satisfied for longer. This is how they help in weight loss.

Nutrients

Vegetables are rich in phytochemicals and special disease-fighting plant pigments, and are low in calories and carbohydrates, with virtually no fat content—avocados and olives being among the very few exceptions.

Servings per day

Include at least 4–6 servings of vegetables a day. One serving of vegetables (cut up) = ½ cup. Try and include at least 50 per cent of the vegetables in raw form, for better energy, good skin and reduced food cravings. Raw vegetables can be included in the form of salads, vegetable juices, raitas and snacks.

Table 4.3: Serving sizes of vegetables

Vegetables	1 serving
Raw leafy vegetables (cut up)	1 cup
Other vegetables (cut up)	1 cup

The wonder foods

Some vegetables might actually help you burn calories when they are consumed as they supposedly take more energy to process and digest than they provide. For example, you will burn about 60 kcal digesting a 15 kcal piece of celery, with a loss of 45 kcal. This is because it is predominantly composed of water, and indigestible fibre in the form of cellulose. Other examples of such vegetables include cabbage, cauliflower, broccoli, berries, turnip, radish, asparagus, grapefruit, cucumber, lettuce and spinach.

The fact is that about 10 per cent of a meal's energy value is used up in digestion and storage of nutrients. This happens when the metabolism is stepped up in the 5 or so hours after finishing a meal. Hence, low-calorie foods require a larger amount of energy to digest compared to the amount of calories they provide. However, such foods should not be considered zero-calorie foods.

Raw versus cooked vegetables

Whether raw vegetables are more beneficial than cooked vegetables has been a subject of debate and much interest. That raw food and cooked food might affect the body differently was proposed as early as the 1930s, when Dr Kouchakoff presented his work on feeding experiments in humans at the First International Congress of Microbiology.

Evidence suggests that cooking vegetables has some harmful effects, as it destroys nutrients and enzymes. However, cooking is indeed beneficial as it not only kills potentially harmful organisms and makes vegetables safe for consumption but also improves the bioavailability of certain nutrients and improves digestibility.

The truth is that vegetables are beneficial in both states—raw and cooked. Cooking vegetables decreases the levels of water-soluble and heat-sensitive nutrients such as vitamin C, vitamin B and folic acid. In fact, it was reported that salad and raw-vegetable consumption has been found to be positively associated with higher levels of these nutrients among adults in the US. The study also showed that the higher levels of these nutrients among salad consumers suggested better absorption.[2] In addition to causing a loss of nutrients and enzyme activity, as well as the formation of harmful by-products called advanced glycation end-products (AGEs), cooking vegetables is likely to raise their glycaemic indices. Therefore, raw vegetables may be more useful for weight-watchers and diabetics.

But there are also positives to cooking vegetables. Besides making them safer, cooking vegetables increases the availability of vitamin A. A study found that heating tomatoes resulted in significantly increased lycopene content and antioxidant activity despite a decrease in vitamin C.[3] So making sure you have a good mix of both raw and

---

2 L.J. Su and L. Arab, 'Salad and Raw Vegetable Consumption and Nutritional Status in the Population: Results from the Third National Health and Nutrition Examination Survey', *Journal of American Dietetic Association* 106, no. 9 (September 2006): 1394–404.

3 Lilli B. Link and John D. Potter, 'Raw versus Cooked Vegetables and Cancer Risk', *Cancer Epidemiology, Biomarkers and Prevention* 13, no. 9 (September 2004): 1422–35.

cooked vegetables in your diet is worthwhile.

Myth: Peas and carrots are fattening.
Fact: Peas and carrots provide good-quality complex carbohydrates, fibre and valuable nutrients. You can happily have them while you are on a weight-loss diet, but remember to include a variety of vegetables.

Myth: Soups and salads are always low in calories.
Fact: Not always. There can be a wide variation depending on what ingredients are used. Soups with only vegetables are low in calories while those with cream and starch may be high in calories. High-calorie soups with a lot of starch, coconut, noodles, pasta, beans, tofu, chicken or other meats can be treated as meal replacements. The same goes for salads with rich dressings.

Myth: Vegetarian diets will help you lose weight more easily.
Fact: This is not necessarily true as vegetarian diets could be high in carbohydrates and low in proteins, and nutrients like vitamin B_{12}, iron and zinc. This can be conterproductive. Well-planned non-vegetarian and vegetarian diets are comparable; what matters is what you include. In fact, a diet that includes high-quality protein through fish, poultry and lean meats is more likely to meet nutrient needs, particularly with regard to vitamin B_{12}, iron and zinc.

Myth: Vegetarians have trouble getting enough protein.
Fact: Vegetarian diets that include proteins from legumes, soy, low-fat dairy, nuts, seeds, whole grains and vegetables in the right proportions can very easily meet protein requirements.

Fruits

Fruits provide high levels of potassium, several minerals and antioxidants, besides making our diet alkaline. While both vegetables and fruits are low in calories, vegetables can be treated as free foods (foods that may be had liberally when attempting weight loss) but excessive amounts of fruit sugar through sweet fruits, dry fruits like raisins, dates, apricots, sultanas, figs, prunes, etc., fruit juices, honey and jaggery interfere with weight loss, particularly for those who are insulin resistant.

In general, fruits are best had fresh and whole. They are great as desserts and snacks. Dry fruits like raisins, dates, figs, apricots, prunes, sultanas, etc. have higher caloric density because they contain concentrated sugar. They make for an excellent choice as sweets, particularly to quell sugar craving. However, use them sparingly and preferably combine them with nuts to ensure they do not upset insulin balance. Excessive intake of dry fruits can also lead to gastrointestinal discomfort like bloating, cramping and loose motions.

Nutrients

Fruits are good sources of nutrients, especially vitamins, minerals (particularly sodium and potassium), phytochemicals and antioxidants.

Servings per day

Substituting grains/cereals with fruits is a wonderful way to lose weight and enhance health. But remember, excessive intake of fruits—that is, more than 2–3 a day—can hinder weight loss. Those with insulin resistance should keep to no more than 1–2 fruits a day and strictly avoid fruit juices. Avoid fruit juices—whether fresh, canned or packed—if you are trying to lose or manage weight. They are low in fibre and have a high glycaemic index. The high glycaemic index of fruits can impair glucose control and may be counterproductive for individuals with insulin resistance or metabolic obesity. If you must have fruit juices, take no more than 100 ml, dilute them with soda or water, or drink a combination of vegetable and fruit juice.

Table 4.4: Serving sizes of commonly consumed fruits

Fruits	1 serving
Most fruits like apples, pears, plums, peaches and oranges (cut up)	½ cup
Fruits with high water content like berries, melons, watermelons, papayas (cut up)	1 cup
Banana	½ (medium)
Grapes	½ cup (16–18 grapes)
Mango	⅓ cup/1 (medium) slice
Strawberries	1 cup (12–14 berries)

Fructose

If you thought going on a fruit diet will help you lose flab, think again! Undisputedly, fruits and vegetables are central to weight-loss diets and good health. However, recent research suggests that excessive intake of sugar from fruits can be harmful. Sugar from fruits, also called fructose, in excessive amounts (>50 gm per day) can be counterproductive for many and may increase the risk of obesity, diabetes and heart disease. A 100 gm apple gives you about 6 gm of fructose and a single serving of a sweetened, carbonated beverage can give you as much as 20 gm of fructose.

Fructose is a simple sugar that is present in fruits, fruit juices, honey, etc., and is responsible for their sweet taste. Besides fruits, a significant source of fructose is table sugar, which is made up of 50 per cent fructose and 50 per cent glucose. Nowadays, fructose is cropping up not just in fruit juices, where it is present naturally, but in all sorts of foods and drinks—from biscuits to ice creams. Fruits and fruit juices are generally perceived as health foods, cholesterol-free and low in calories and fat. They are in fact a disguised form of fructose. For those who believe that fresh fruit juice is a good alternative to the canned or packed versions, the truth is that it may contain about 25 gm of fructose per cup. Sweetened beverages and fruit juices contribute significantly to high fructose intake in urban diets worldwide, leading to the piling up of extra kilos without our realizing it, and in part explains the growing epidemics of obesity, diabetes, heart disease.

Unlike other sugars such as glucose, fructose in excessive quantities is associated with insulin resistance, leading to metabolic syndrome and associated complications. Individuals who are particularly vulnerable to high fructose levels include those who are overweight and insulin resistant or diabetic. According to recent research, the rate of fructose intake correlates closely with the rate of diabetes worldwide.[4]

Fructose intake causes fat to accumulate in the blood and liver. Instead of being used immediately for energy, the fructose is readily converted into triglycerides by the liver. According to the National Institute of Health (United States), the growing incidence of gout

---

4 R.J. Johnson and others, 'Hypothesis: Could Excessive Fructose Intake and Uric Acid Cause Type 2 Diabetes?', *Endocrine Reviews* 30, no. 1 (February 2009): 96–119.

due to high uric acid levels also coincides with a substantial increase in the consumption of soft drinks and fructose. Most of us do not know that fructose can be listed in the ingredients under a variety of names—the most common being high-fructose corn syrup (HFCS). It has been reported that adding a single HFCS-sweetened soft drink to each meal for 10 weeks significantly increases blood fat levels which can eventually lead to fatty liver, pre-diabetes or metabolic syndrome.

Studies done as early as the 1950s have reported that diets high in sugar, especially fructose, can rapidly induce features of metabolic syndrome.[5] Researchers found that when overweight individuals were fed equal calories from glucose and fructose, both sugars caused about the same degree of weight gain, but an important difference in the nature of these gains was evident. Individuals in the 'fructose' group gained more fat in their abdominal area;[6] this is known to elevate the risk of diabetes and heart disease to a greater degree than fat stored elsewhere in the body.

Conversely, those with metabolic syndrome, fatty liver and high levels of uric acid have been found to have a history of significantly greater fructose intake. Diets with fructose levels as low as 15–25 per cent can illustrate the ability of fructose to induce insulin resistance. Recently, one of my clients, who came to me looking for a diet to manage his excess weight, was also concerned about his high uric acid

---

5 Ibid.

6 T. Nakagawa and others, 'A Casual Role for Uric Acid in Fructose-induced Metabolic Syndrome', *American Journal of Physiology—Renal Physiology* 290, no. 3 (March 2006): F625–31; S. Reungjui and others, 'Thiazide Diuretics Exacerbate Fructose-induced Metabolic Syndrome', *Journal of American Society of Nephrology* 18, no. 10 (October 2007): 2724–31.

levels. While telling me about his average day's diet, he mentioned that he liked fruits a lot and was consuming about 5–6 fruits a day; it was then that I realized the reason behind his high uric acid levels. Also, when we carried out his body composition analysis, it was found that his abdominal fat (visceral fat) was way above the normal range. I explained to him then the reason for his excess weight, high uric acid levels and high visceral fat. It has been rightly said that too much of anything is not good, and the same stands true for fruits too.

There is an urgent need for increased public awareness of the risks associated with high fructose consumption, and greater efforts should be made to curb the addition of packaged foods with high-fructose additives to one's diet. So, next time you go on that 'fruit diet', watch your portions. A prudent approach to the intake of fruits must be maintained. In general, enjoy the pleasures of sweets within limits. Soft drinks, sweetened drinks, punches, cocktails and fruit juices, which contain empty calories, must be replaced with water, plain soda, coconut water, low-fat milk and vegetable juices.

Hidden sources of fructose

These include sugar, honey, jaggery, molasses, brown sugar, cane sugar, corn sweetener, corn or agave syrup, sucrose, laevulose and maple syrup.

HFCS (a combination of 50 per cent fructose and 50 per cent glucose), a sweetener used commercially by the food industry, is a major ingredient in soft drinks, desserts, fruit yogurts, cereals, health bars, ice creams, biscuits, pastries and processed foods. Food manufacturers prefer to use HFCS in place of sugar for several reasons. It is cheap, easy to use and more stable than simple sugar; it also increases the shelf life and improves the texture of products. It is used in cereal bars and biscuits to make them chewy, to thicken ice creams and yogurt drinks, reduce crystallization in frozen products and improve the colour of baked products. The introduction of HFCS in the 1970s has resulted in a 30 per cent increase in total fructose intake in the last 20 years through soft drinks, fruit drinks and juices, and processed foods, and has been associated with a significant increase in the rates of obesity and diabetes.

Fruit juices versus vegetable juices

Having a lot of fruits or fruit juices can affect those with insulin resistance or metabolic obesity and will certainly affect weight loss. Ideally, fruits should be consumed before or after exercise if you are on a diet. Vegetable juices, on the other hand, constitute a filling meal by themselves and will help with weight loss. Bottle gourd (doodhi, lauki or ghia) juice is a low-calorie, low-carbohydrate beverage with moderate potassium and fibre content. Its good satiety makes it useful for weight-watchers, diabetics, hypertensives and heart patients. Instead of a fruit juice you could look at having a mixed-vegetable juice (cucumber, carrot and/or tomato, boosted with beetroot, celery and/or amla work well) with a dash of some fruit if you wish, when trying to lose weight.

> Myth: Fruit diets can make you lose weight.
> Fact: Yes, they can. However, as too much of anything can be counterproductive, stick to about 2–3 fruits a day. Often, people think that by going on a fruit and juice diet, they will lose weight quickly. This might be counterproductive for people who have insulin resistance

or a strong family history of diabetes. Fruit juices are not recommended during weight loss, as fruit sugar (fructose) can worsen insulin resistance/metabolism.

Myth: Melons and watermelons help lose weight.
Fact: Melons and watermelons have high water content and glycaemic index; they can be very sweet too. Large quantities can cause excessive fructose intake which may interfere with weight loss.

Low-fat dairy and dairy products

These include skimmed milk, low-fat yogurt, cottage cheese and cheese. Dairy products along with calcium and special fatty acids like CLAs (see section on CLAs, p. 50) also promote fat loss, help in obesity management and regulate blood pressure. CLAs are also known to possess anti-cancer properties.

Nutrients

They contain first-class proteins because they contain all the essential amino acids that are very good for your body. They are rich in calcium, magnesium and phosphorus which are bone-building nutrients, and also provide vitamins A, D, B_2 (riboflavin), and CLAs.

Servings per day

One serving provides roughly 70–80 kcal. Include 2–3 servings of low-fat dairy a day. For obesity management, 1–2 servings a day must be included. For those who are lactose intolerant, yogurt and soy milk are good alternatives.

Table 4.5: Serving sizes of commonly consumed dairy products

Dairy product	**1 serving**
Cheese	2 slices
Cottage cheese	½ cup/½ deck of cards
Feta cheese	¼ cup/3 dice
Milk	1 cup
Yogurt	1 cup

For the dairy intolerant

Dairy-intolerant individuals need not despair as benefits similar to those gained by dairy consumption can be obtained by including calcium-rich foods like soy and soy products (tofu, miso, soy milk, etc.), green leafy vegetables, seaweeds, sesame seeds, flaxseeds, sunflower seeds, poppy seeds, almonds and other nuts, finger millet (ragi) and amaranth.

The calcium weight-loss effect

Dairy products are great for us but unfortunately they are also high in fat. However, studies have shown that calcium can actually help you get rid of fat in your body. We all know that fat is something we need to cut down on, if we are counting calories. Researchers stumbled upon the calcium weight-loss effect by accident in the 1980s when studying the relationship between diet and blood pressure.[7] The effect remains controversial, but dozens of studies have added evidence that it is legitimate, at least in the case of people who are

7 Jill Fullerton-Smith, *The Truth about Food* (London: Bloomsbury, 2007), 63.

already overweight. A study reported that people who consumed low-fat dairy had lower body fat percentages compared to their counterparts.

> Myth: The fat content of milk may be reduced by adding water.
> Fact: If water is added to milk, all other nutrients, along with fat, get diluted. Skimming the fatty layer is the best way to remove fat from milk at home, as this ensures that the other nutrients are retained. Alternatively, choose double-toned milk or skimmed milk with less than 1 per cent fat.

> Myth: Adolescents should not be given milk as this will cause weight gain during their teenage years.
> Fact: The most damaging consequence of insufficient milk intake during childhood and adolescence is dwarfism and weight gain. Other potentially adverse consequences of avoiding dairy include an involuntary increase in sugar intake through sweetened beverages to compensate for inadequate energy intake. During childhood, at least 2–3 servings of dairy a day must be emphasized.

> Myth: Low-fat frozen yogurt may be counted under 'dairy'.
> Fact: While low-fat yogurt is a rich source of dairy and calcium, it is more often than not also loaded with sugars. Hence, it is better counted under 'desserts' and is OK to be had as an occasional treat.

Myth: Cottage cheese and cheese should not be had while attempting weight loss.
Fact: Cottage cheese and cheese may indeed be had while attempting weight loss, as long as you control the portions. Thirty–fifty gm of cottage cheese or 2 slices of cheese are equivalent to 1 serving of low-fat dairy. You need not make cottage cheese at home, if good-quality cottage cheese is available off the shelf.

Meat, fish, chicken and eggs

These are your primary sources of first-class proteins and fat. They are also rich in easily absorbable iron (haem iron). This food group also includes cured and processed meats.

Nutrients

Eggs, including the yolk, are highly nutritious and provide excellent proteins with few calories. They provide several valuable nutrients like vitamin A, beta-carotene, zinc and B vitamins. In other words, they are nutrient packed and help keep you full for long.

Fish and shellfish provide special protective fats called omega-3 fats (see section on PUFAs, p. 49). Omega-3 fats in fish help in weight management, protect us from inflammatory conditions like heart disease, arthritis and asthma, improve immunity and brain function as well as regulate blood pressure.

The fat and cholesterol content in lean red meat is comparable to that in poultry and fish. Meat contains about 20–23 per cent protein and varying amounts of fat (5–30 per cent); however, the nature of fat differs. Red-meat fat is more saturated than poultry fat. The maturity of the animal affects the meat texture and fat content. Some cuts have higher levels of fat than others, and huge variations in fat content exist among meats. For example, lamb is not marbled like beef. Meat from the shoulder, shank and neck is leaner compared to meat from the breast. Since much of the fat is located outside of the meat, it can be trimmed before cooking. Organ meats such as liver and kidney are relatively low in fat but high in cholesterol, and should be eaten less often, no more than once a month.

Meat is an excellent source of vitamin B complex, especially vitamin B_{12}, niacin, zinc and bioavailable haem iron. Meat protein is high quality, that is, it provides all the essential amino acids that cannot be made by the body. Meat is also a source of CLAs, which have been found to be useful in the reduction of cholesterol and body fat (see section on CLAs, p. 50) and, in addition, may possess potentially anti-carcinogenic properties.

Accumulating scientific evidence suggests that lean red meat is a healthy and beneficial component of any well-balanced diet as long as it is fat trimmed and consumed as a part of a varied diet. However, what is important is to assess the appropriate portion and fat content of meat and the quality of diet in general. The American Institute for Cancer Research (AICR) and the American Dietetic Association (ADA) recommend limiting red-meat intake to 250 gm a week. The usual amount per serving is about 120 gm with little or no bone. In other words, if you eat lean red meat once or twice a week as a part of a healthy diet, you have nothing to fear.

Servings per day

Half–one and a half servings a day of any of the above-mentioned meats, as long as you regularly steer clear of cured and processed meats, are adequate. Each serving provides 150–170 kcal. An egg a day is safe for most. People with high blood cholesterol, and heart disease, should limit their egg intake to 3–4 eggs per week. Fish should be consumed at least twice a week and chicken and lean red meat may be eaten twice a week as well, always with lots of vegetables. Non-vegetarians should try to restrict lean meat to only one meal a day.

Table 4.6: Serving sizes of eggs and commonly consumed meats

Food type	1 serving
Chicken	100 gm/1 deck of cards
Eggs	2
Fish	100 gm/1 chequebook
Lean meat	100 gm/1 deck of cards

Note: Cured and processed meats like sausages, salami, ham and bacon are high in fat and salt. The fat content of such meats can exceed 40 per cent. Some kebabs like seekh, kakori and galouti can be exceptionally high in fat. They are best restricted to treats.

> Myth: Eggs are high in cholesterol and should therefore be avoided.
>
> Fact: An egg contains nearly 215 mg cholesterol—surely the intake of a single yolk could exhaust the entire day's limit of 300 mg cholesterol! However, studies have found no significant correlation between the consumption of eggs and heart disease. A study by the University of Surrey reported that people who consume 1 or more eggs a day are no more at risk of developing heart disease than non-egg eaters.[8] Britain's Foods Standards Agency says there

8 J. Gray and B. Griffin, 'Eggs and Dietary Cholesterol—Dispelling the Myth', *Nutrition Bulletin* 34, no. 1 (March 2009): 66–70.

is no limit to eating eggs if they are part of a balanced diet. As a part of a healthy diet, egg cholesterol seems to have little impact on blood cholesterol levels. Several studies have shown that regular egg consumption induces little to modest changes in blood cholesterol in people with both normal and high cholesterol levels. People with high blood cholesterol/heart disease should limit their egg intake to 3–4 eggs per week as part of a healthy diet. For everyone else, an egg a day is safe. With only 75 kcal, eggs provide excellent-quality protein. Packed with nutrients and high satiety, they are ideal when attempting weight loss.

Myth: Fish and shellfish are high in cholesterol.
Fact: Edible marine fish and shellfish such as clams, mussels, scallops, oysters, lobsters and shrimp represent an important, highly nutritious food source. They are low in saturated fat and calories and are a good source of protein, iron, vitamin B_{12}, iodine, phosphorus, zinc and copper. Fish and fish oil are particularly rich in omega-3 fatty acids, which help reduce inflammation in conditions like arthritis as well as the risk of blood clot formation, thus offering protection against heart attacks. Grilled, baked or broiled fish (instead of fried) works well as part of a healthy weight-loss plan.

Nuts and seeds

Nuts include almonds, walnuts, cashews, pistachios, peanuts, pine nuts, macadamia nuts, hazelnuts, etc. Seeds include sesame seeds, flaxseeds, sunflower seeds, pumpkin seeds, cucumber seeds, melon seeds, chia seeds, etc.

Many people believe that nuts are high in cholesterol and bad for the heart, while others believe that they are bad for weight loss as they are high in calories. Both these beliefs are untrue. Nuts and seeds have a very low glycaemic index and play a vital role in weight management. Their high satiety value makes them an ideal snack for weight-watchers. They offer the easiest way to relieve hunger pangs and help prevent food cravings by regulating blood sugar levels and providing vital nutrients.

Nutrients

Nuts and seeds are nutrient-packed foods and free of cholesterol. They are rich in high-quality fat, heart-healthy poly- and monounsaturated fats, omega-3 fats, fibre, magnesium, vitamin E and phytochemicals like flavonoids (antioxidants which serve as disease-fighting chemicals). They are also a good source of plant protein, B vitamins, and minerals like zinc, copper and selenium. They are one of the best sources of arginine, an amino acid that serves as the precursor of nitric oxide synthesis. They contain small amounts of folate and are low in carbohydrates. Flavonoids help protect blood vessels and cells from damage, reduce the risk of heart disease and cancer, and delay ageing. Copper prevents high blood pressure. Magnesium and potassium prevent high blood pressure, arrhythmia and heart attacks. Fibre helps improve high blood cholesterol, blood sugar levels in diabetics, as well as blood pressure. Folate helps check the build-up of homocysteine (a kind of amino acid associated with heart disease) in blood. Good-quality fat and phytosterols help reduce blood cholesterol levels.

Serving

Include a handful a day. Each serving gives about 100–120 kcal. Nuts are nutrient-dense snacks; they help curb cravings and act as natural appetite suppressants. Remember, they too have calories, so do not overdo their intake.

Table 4.7: Serving sizes of commonly consumed nuts and seeds

Nuts and seeds	1 serving (30 gm)
Almonds (shelled)	23 pcs
Cashews	16 pcs
Peanuts	28 pcs
Pistachios (unshelled)	45 pcs
Seeds	3 tbsp
Walnut halves (shelled)	14 pcs

Myth: As nuts are high in cholesterol and calories, they should be avoided while attempting weight loss.

Fact: Nuts certainly are high in calories but have no cholesterol. They have several advantages with regard to weight loss. They are low in carbohydrates and loaded with good-quality fat, protein and nutrients that help fight cravings, making them excellent snacks, if taken in moderation.

Fats and oils

Fats are an essential part of our diet. Apart from being present in nuts, seeds and some fruits and vegetables like coconut and avocado, they are also found in butter, clarified butter (ghee) and an array of oils.

Nutrients

They provide essential fatty acids, which cannot be made by the body, and serve as an energy reserve. Fats are necessary for the absorption of fat-soluble vitamins including vitamins A, D, E and K.

Servings per day

For a 2000 kcal diet, 1 serving should include 4–5 tsp daily. One tsp provides about 45 kcal.

A combination of oils is preferred over a single oil to balance the nutritional requirements of PUFAs, MUFAs and SFAs, all of which are good for you. A prudent choice would be a combination of mustard, canola, rice bran and sesame oils along with moderate amounts of butter, clarified butter or unprocessed coconut oil. Extra virgin or virgin olive oil, along with the above, makes for an excellent choice. We need to watch the quality of fat in addition to the quantity of fat. The best fats can be obtained from nuts, seeds, fatty fish, avocado, and coconut, olive and cold-pressed oils. MUFA-rich oils like olive oil, mustard oil, seasame oil and canola oil help in reducing belly fat.

Trans fats: A no-no

Trans fats are a by-product of hydrogenation—a process that turns fats which are liquid at room temperature into fats that are solid at room temperature, like margarine and shortenings. Approximately 70 per cent of all fat used in processed foods such as crackers, cookies, pastries, cakes and fried foods is hydrogenated. In India, trans fats entered our diets around the 1960s and early 1970s in the form of vanaspati and then later through bakery products that used margarines and shortenings. Reheated oil also contains trans fats.

Trans fats have been linked to most modern diseases, including cardiovascular disease, cancer, obesity, diabetes, and compromised immunity. Although the harmful effects of hydrogenated fats and trans fats have been well established by numerous scientific studies, they continue to be a part of our diet, thanks to skewed labelling, smart marketing and 'half-truth' advertisements. Products with tags such as 'cholesterol-free', '100 per cent natural', 'no animal fat', 'low in saturated fat', 'lite' and 'sugar-free' are usually loaded with trans fats. So harmful are trans fats that health and nutrition experts have zero tolerance for them.

Labelling laws, until recently, did not require trans fats to be mentioned separately and they were grouped under 'saturated fat content'. This meant that labels could simply say 'low saturated fat' but could still contain trans fats. Food manufacturers could consequently increase the content of trans fats in their products while decreasing the amount of beneficial saturated fats.

Since 2006, the US Food and Drug Administration (USFDA) has made it mandatory for food manufacturers in the US to reveal the levels of trans fat in packed foods separately; these guidelines suggest that the total trans fat content in a food product should not be more than 1 per cent of the total calories, that is, approximately 2 gm daily. However, adhering to such standards may be difficult and for all practical purposes foods containing less than 0.5 gm trans fat per serving are able to list 'zero trans fats' on their 'nutrition facts' panel. These standards apply only to packaged food and not to foods served in restaurants. However, as consumers begin to see nutrition labels listing trans fat quantities and continue to hear more about trans fats through the media and other sources, they may begin to seek more information about trans fat content even in food served in restaurants. We hope to see such interventions against trans fats in our country soon!

Many products like trans fat–free margarines and bread spreads have appeared in the last decade in Europe, and are making an entry into India as well. The two questions these raise are:

1. Are they really 'trans fat–free'?
2. Are they healthier options to conventional natural fats like butter?

My view is that while the production method may well be healthier, it is always safer to go for the more natural options.

Refined versus cold-pressed oils

Based on the mode of extraction, oils can be categorized as refined and cold-pressed; the latter is also known as kachi ghani. Refined oils are produced by heating oils at very high temperatures (more than 200°C). Heat destroys all the essential fats, vitamins and antioxidants present in fats. Refined oils are also subjected to chemical processing and hydrogenation which further causes the formation of harmful chemical compounds including trans fats. This makes oils almost 'nutritionally naked'. High heat refining can cause the formation of 'new chemical compounds' which are mutagenic or carcinogenic.

Cold-pressed oils are extracted at room temperature without employing chemicals or high temperatures. This retains their natural goodness. Olive, mustard and sesame are some of the commonly used cold-pressed oils in traditional households and are also commercially available now.

Myth: Cooking in olive oil is less calorific.
Fact: Olive oil has the same number of calories as any other oil. But since it has high density, you require lesser amounts.

Myth: Margarine is less fattening than butter.
Fact: There is no significant difference between the two in terms of calories. Hydrogenated margarine is rich in harmful trans fats. Newer margarines may be better, with 'no trans fats' and added phytochemicals, but only marginally.

Sugars

According to WHO recommendations, less than 10 per cent of our total calories should come from free sugars. Excessive calories from free sugars can contribute to increased cravings, insulin imbalance, weight gain, increase in triglycerides (blood fats) and dental problems. The ironic thing about sugars is that the more you eat the more you need.

Grains/cereals, starches, honey, molasses, fruits and fruit juices are sugars in disguise and hence it's advisable to get your sugars from these rather than have added sugars or pure-sugar products such as soft drinks, etc. Molasses, honey and jaggery are better as sweeteners from a health perspective but affect weight in the same way. Sugar substitutes should be kept to a minimum.

Nutrients

These are high in carbohydrates and calories and low in nutrients.

Servings per day

Sugars and sweets must be treated as discretionary foods. While you need not give them up entirely, be smart about how you eat them and in what quantity. Giving children less sugar is worthwhile as the palate can be trained early in life. High sugar intake is not recommended for anyone—even if you are not diabetic or overweight.

> Myth: Honey, brown sugar and molasses are better than sugar and are OK to consume when trying to manage weight.
> Fact: They contain a similar amount of carbohydrates and calories, and therefore have the same effect on weight. Nutritionally speaking, molasses, gur, unrefined sugar (shakkar) and honey are certainly healthier options.

> Myth: 'Sugar-free' labels ensure that the food in question is healthy and safe.
> Fact: Look around and you see supermarket shelves stacked with 'sugar-free' chocolates, jams, cookies, drinks and much more. Do 'sugar-free' options really deliver what they promise? People often associate 'sugar-free' foods with lower calories, and thereby consider them beneficial for diabetics and weight-watchers. This may not always be the case. 'Sugar-free' foods may be loaded with fats, refined cereals (white flour, starch, etc.) and even hidden sugars (fructose, maltitol, etc.) which when eaten in large quantities can have detrimental effects on health. Read labels carefully when going in for 'sugar-free' products.

Myth: Products that belong to 'healthy-eating' ranges are the most beneficial when trying to lose weight.
Fact: This might be the case for some products, but not all. Many 'healthy-eating' products focus mainly on cutting down the fat content, and pay little attention to the levels of carbohydrates and the quality and quantity of fats and nutrients.

Myth: 'Low-fat' or 'non-fat' equals no calories.
Fact: Many low-fat or non-fat foods may still have a lot of calories. Often these foods have extra sugar, refined flour or starch thickeners to make them taste better. These ingredients add calories from carbohydrates which may lead to weight gain.

Myth: 'Cholesterol-free' labels ensure that the product is 'trouble-free' and will not affect your health, weight or heart.
Fact: Products marked 'cholesterol-free' may not contain cholesterol but may contain other harmful fats like trans fats and undesirable ingredients. For example, fried snacks like namkeens, wafers and vegetarian snacks might be prepared in hydrogenated oils.

Reading food labels

Shifting away from the traditional home-cooked foods, we are now consuming more convenience, packaged and ready-to-eat foods. Some of these foods may be healthy while some may not be so. Understanding the food labels and the nutrition information given on food packages can help us decide easily as to which food to choose.

Further, the correct interpretation of the labels is important as sometimes the nutrition claims can be misleading and may highlight what is not naturally present in a food product and is good rather than what is present in it and is harmful.

What to look for on the label

1. The ingredients list provides the list of food items that are present in the packaged product. Usually, ingredients (except water) are listed in the descending order by weight. The first ingredient in the list is the one found in the greatest amount, and the last ingredient is the one found in the least amount.
2. The nutrition information panel gives the nutrition information of the products. Learning to read food labels can help us understand and interpret the information in a meaningful way.
   a. Per 100 gm: 100 gm is a useful standard to compare products on the basis of their nutritional composition.
   b. Calories: A product is considered low calorie if it provides 40 kcal or less per serving.
   c. Fat: Besides the total amount of fat, it is important to check the amount of saturated fat and trans fats in a product. A product is considered low fat if it provides 3 gm of fat or less per serving and fat-free if it has less than ½ gm fat per serving. Fat may be hidden as vegetable fat, vegetable oil, coconut oil, cream, sour cream, di- or monoglycerides, lard, mayonnaise, palm oil, shortenings, tallow or toasted nuts.
   d. Cholesterol: A product may claim to be a low-cholesterol product if it has less than 20 mg cholesterol.
   e. Sodium: Choose products with less than 140 mg of sodium

per serving. Sodium may be disguised as baking powder, baking soda, booster, hydrolysed vegetable, hydrolysed meat, meat/yeast extracts, sodium, monosodium glutamate (MSG), sodium metabisulphite, rock salt, sea salt, stock cube, stock powder and/or vegetable/herb salt (for example, oregano, garlic, onion, celery).

f. Sugar refers to the amount of carbohydrate present as sugar. It includes both natural as well as added sugar. A product may include sugar in the form of sucrose as well as other sugars like fructose, dextrose, dextrine, malitol and HFCS. A product may claim to be sugar-free if it has less than ½ gm of sugar per serving.
g. Sugars may be disguised as dextrose, sucrose, lactose, fructose, glucose, golden syrup, corn syrup, maple syrup, brown sugar, raw sugar, invert sugar, molasses, saccharides, modified carbohydrate, malt, malt extract, maltose, maltodextrins, mannitol, sorbitol, xylitol and/or honey.
h. Fibre: Choose products with high fibre content. A product with a fibre content >5 gm per 100 gm is considered a high-fibre product.

3. The 'per cent daily value' that is mentioned on some of the food labels is based on the recommended dietary intake and is calculated for a 2000 kcal diet. A product may say that it is a:
   a. Good source of any nutrient if it provides at least 10 per cent of the daily value of a particular vitamin or nutrient per serving.
   b. High in any nutrient if it provides 20 per cent or more of the daily value of the specified nutrient per serving.
   c. Healthy if the following are true in its case: it is low fat, has low saturated fat, less than 480 mg sodium, less than 95 mg

cholesterol and at least 10 per cent of the daily value of vitamins A and C, iron, protein, calcium and fibre.

Nutrition claims can help one choose healthy food products; however, they can at times be misleading too. With this, label reading has become all the more important.

✚ ADDING IT ALL UP

When you put food on a plate, train your eye to divide it up on the basis of food groups. You should also start to think about how much of what you should be eating. The key to losing weight correctly is to eat foods from all food groups but in the right proportions since almost all of these foods have beneficial properties. Remember to include the following:

1. Generous amounts of vegetables, fruits and water.
2. Moderate amounts of protein-rich foods like low-fat dairy, lean meat, pulses and legumes, and nuts and seeds.
3. Limited amounts of carbohydrates, oils, fats, alcohol and high-sugar, high-fat foods.
4. Occasional intake of junk foods, pies, puddings, desserts and celebration foods.

The key to losing weight is to limit sugars and excessive grains/cereals, and have beneficial foods like vegetables, pulses, fruits, low-fat dairy, lean meats, and good fats through nuts and seeds, with a special focus on raw vegetables, fruits and sprouts. But how do we use these principles and actually plan our day-to-day eating? Let's move to the next chapter.

5

THE DIET PLANS

✚ THE DOCTOR SAYS

Let's summarize the previous chapters. The key to losing weight is to eat fewer calories than your normal intake and manage the right proportion of calories, proteins and fats. However to lose weight effectively and in a healthy way, you shouldn't expect to lose more than 1 kg a week on an average; if you are insulin resistant or have metabolic obesity, this figure should be halved.

You should not give up eating foods arbitrarily or based on common conceptions of what is considered 'healthy' and what is not. What you do need to do is lower your intake of foods from some food groups (in particular, grains/cereals), fats and sugars, and up your intake of vegetables and fruits. Low-fat dairy, pulses, nuts and seeds are also vital.

When I prescribe diets to my clients, no one questions my curtailing of sugars and fats. We all know that too much of these aren't good for us. But there is always surprise about how much grains/cereals I allow them. By now you know what I feel about grains/cereals—that while they are good for us, we tend to consume them in amounts far greater than what we need. Most people fill their stomach with grains/cereals and they fear that on the diets I prescribe, they will be permanently hungry.

Wrong. Load up on your vegetables and remember to put in low-fat dairy, pulses and other protein-rich foods—they are often filling foods with high satiety value. But how do you put all this together? And isn't all this too much thinking? Relax—you've done all your thinking in the previous chapters. Now it's time to act.

Before we begin

Before we begin, I want to put forth a few words of caution. Many of my clients give up and go off track completely, if they deviate from the plans. Do not begin with an 'all-or-nothing' mindset. Remember, no one is expected to be perfect at all times. Context, moderation, balance and variety are the golden words in diet management. So keep the following principles in mind as you begin your new eating plans.

Context

Very often people check if they can eat a particular food while they are on their weight-loss plan: 'Can I eat a mango?', 'Can I have a dosa?', 'Can I have a drink?', etc. Well, the answer is yes, but in context—it all depends on what you have eaten earlier and what you propose to eat later. In other words, no food is strictly prohibited. You must learn to make it a part of your diet without it conflicting with your goals. Remember, for 'indulgence foods', the frequency, amounts and context are important.

Moderation

No food is good or bad; what matters is the amount you take. When you proclaim foods 'off limits', you are setting up a rule just waiting to be broken. Portion control is a key to healthy eating. A small portion of dessert rather than the entire helping will be a good idea and is unlikely to conflict with your goals.

Balance

There may be days when moderation or portion control fails. You go through the entire dessert and feel terribly guilty. The principle of balance helps you undo the damage and lighten the next meal to compensate for the previous one, and this will ensure that you do not mess up your goals. Balance may also be achieved by engaging in physical activity, by walking that extra mile. Balance can be anticipatory or retrospective. Anticipatory balance refers to the following: if you are likely to overeat later in the day, under-eat or lighten your meal before that. Retrospective balance implies damage control after eating more than you should have.

Variety

Variety is indeed the spice of life. How many different foods do you eat every day: ten–fifteen? Would it surprise you that one of Japan's dietary guidelines suggests eating thirty different foods each day? Variety ensures that your body gets all the nutrients it needs. Make sure that you include foods from all the food groups, and maintain variety within food groups. For example, an apple is rich in vitamin E and poor in vitamin C while an orange is rich in vitamin C and poor in vitamin E. Eating both ensures that you get enough of both the nutrients. Eating a variety of foods prevents food sensitivities. For instance, within the 'grains/cereal' food group, eating a variety of grains is better than subsisting only on rice or wheat.

So now you are armed with knowledge about food groups, nutrients and the four golden rules of weight management. You are ready to begin your journey towards weight loss.

The half-plate rule

First, always pre-plate your food. Put all the food that you want to eat on your plate in one go, so that you can see exactly what you are eating. This not only makes you ensure you control your portions but also that you have the right amount of food from each food group. Research shows that those who plate all their food instead of going for seconds and thirds eat 14 per cent less.[1] The traditional Indian thali or the Japanese bento box are great representations of this.

Now, aim to keep to the 'half-plate' rule. Half your plate should be full of vegetables. Divide the rest of it with foods from the other food groups and treat grains/cereals as a side dish, not a filler. Modest amounts of protein should be included in the form of pulses, dals, nuts, low-fat dairy, eggs, lean meat, chicken and fish.

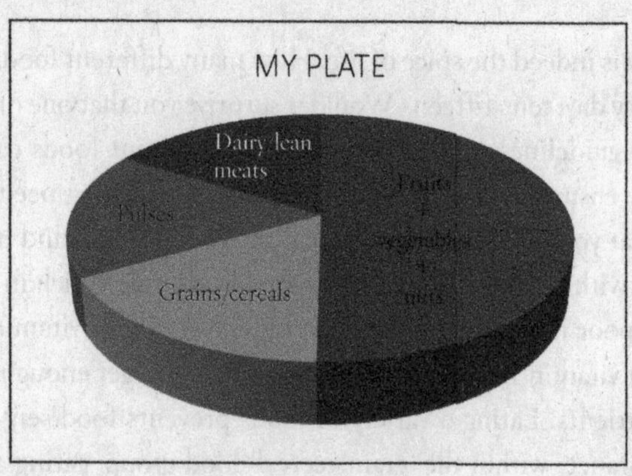

1 Brian Wansink, 'The Forgotten Food' in *Mindless Eating: Why We Eat More Than We Think* (New Delhi: Hay House, 2009), 56.

If you are aware of your required caloric intake, start by making a note of how many servings of each food group you require in a day. If not, proceed to the diet plans and recommendations, and plan your diet accordingly. If I had to summarize, I would simply say: use the half-plate rule, minimize sugars, reduce your current grains/cereals intake to half and fill up on vegetables. Also include at least 2–3 servings of good protein through pulses, low-fat dairy, lean meats and good fats through nuts and seeds.

The basic diet plan

Here are some food group servings with which to begin your diet. Remember, before you begin, you need to calculate the amount of calories you need for your weight; if you are going on a weight-loss diet, subtract 500 kcal from your daily caloric intake. If you are trying to maintain your weight, then adhere to the required caloric amount.

The vegetarian diet plan

Table 5.1: The vegetarian diet plan

Food groups	**Number of servings per day**					**Examples**
Calories (kcal)	**800**	**1000**	**1200**	**1400**	**1600**	**1 serving**
Grains/cereals	1	2	2	3	4	3 tbsp flour 3 cups popcorn 1 slice bread 1 cup puffed cereal/namkeen (roasted)

Food groups	**Number of servings per day**					**Examples**
Calories (kcal)	**800**	**1000**	**1200**	**1400**	**1600**	**1 serving**
						1 chapatti ½ cup rice/pasta/ noodles (cooked)
Pulses	1	2	2	2	3	3–4 (medium) squares dhokla 3 tbsp gram flour 2 (medium) vadas 2 (medium) cheelas 1 cup sprouts 1 cup liquid dal/ pulse/kadhi/ sambar/soy nuggets
Low-fat dairy	1	2	3	3	3	1 cup milk/yogurt ½ cup cottage cheese
Vegetables	4 or more	4 or more	4 or more	4 or more	5 or more	½ cup (cut up)
Fruits	1	2	2	3	3	½–1 cup (cut up)
Nuts and seeds	1	1	1	1	1	1 handful
Fat	2	2	2	2	2	4–5 tsp (for a 2000 kcal diet)
Sugar	1	2	3	4	4	Must be treated as a discretionary food

Note: For serving sizes, see all tables in Chapter 4.

The non-vegetarian diet plan

Table 5.2: The non-vegetarian diet plan

Food groups	**Number of servings per day**					**Examples**
Calories (kcal)	**800**	**1000**	**1200**	**1400**	**1600**	**1 serving**
Grains/cereals	1	2	2	3	4	3 tbsp flour 3 cups popcorn 1 slice bread 1 cup puffed cereal/namkeen (roasted) 1 chapatti ½ cup rice/pasta/noodles (cooked)
Pulses	1	1	1	1	1	3–4 (medium) squares dhokla 3 tbsp gram flour 2 (medium) vadas 2 (medium) cheelas 1 cup sprouts 1 cup liquid dal/pulse//kadhi/sambar/soy nuggets
Lean meats, chicken, fish	1	1	1	1	1	100 gm lean meat/chicken/fish
Eggs	1	1	1	1	1	2 eggs

Food groups	Number of servings per day					Examples
Calories (kcal)	**800**	**1000**	**1200**	**1400**	**1600**	**1 serving**
Low-fat dairy	1	2	2	2	2	1 cup milk/yogurt ½ cup cottage cheese
Vegetables	3 or more	3 or more	4 or more	4 or more	5 or more	½ cup (cut up)
Fruits	1	2	2	3	3	½ –1 cup (cut up)
Nuts and seeds	½	½	½	1	1	1 handful
Fat	1	1	2	2	2	4–5 tsp (for a 2000 kcal diet)
Sugar	1	2	2	4	4	Must be treated as a discretionary food

Note: For serving sizes, see all tables in Chapter 4.

Meal plans

This section illustrates how you can combine different food groups which can help you plan your diet with or without grains/cereals. Remember, these are only some options; this can be done in a hundred different ways according to your preferences—which means that your diet can be truly customized and adapted to any situation. Keep the following in mind:

1. Choose to consume grains/cereals between 8 a.m. and 7 p.m., ideally divided between two meals.
2. Since grain/cereal servings are limited, ideally, choose to eat your grains/cereals at times of peak hunger or pre- or post-exercise. For most people, peak-hunger time is between 5 p.m. and 7 p.m.

Like currency, you may exchange one grain/cereal for another. For example, if you want to have pizza in place of chapatti, you may go in for 2–3 slices of thin-crust pizza instead of a chapatti. (See section on grains/cereals, p. 56.)

3. Taper off grains/cereals—avoid or reduce portions of grains/cereals if you eat dinner late.
4. In the main meals try to include foods from no more than three food groups, and in the smaller meals or snacks, include foods from no more than two food groups. This will help you keep things on track.
5. For main meals, try to aim for up to two protein-rich foods, that is, pulses, dals, dairy, egg, fish, chicken, etc., and combine them with raw or cooked vegetables, fruits or grains/cereals in sensible ways.

For example:

1. Sprouts/dal + salad
2. Milk + fruit
3. Cottage cheese + chapatti
4. Cottage cheese/egg + salad
5. Fish + rice
6. Chicken + vegetables

Breakfast

While breakfast is one of the most important meals of the day, the aim is to pack in maximum nutrition while maintaining a modest number of calories. A high-nutrient breakfast, apart from having a low glycaemic index, will keep you feeling full and energized through the morning as against a large breakfast loaded with carbohydrates and grains which may make you sleepy and lethargic within a couple of hours. In my experience, clients differ significantly in their need to eat in the morning. For those who do not have an exceptionally large appetite and have desk/sedentary jobs, a grain-/cereal-free option or a limited grain/cereal option is more appropriate. Also, for those who are active and on the move, like teachers and children, a breakfast with grains/cereals is recommended.

Depending on your requirements, any of the following options could be chosen for a good breakfast. You may also make your own combinations, depending on your likes and dislikes.

Table 5.3: The breakfast meal plan with options

Options	With grain/cereal (approx. 200 kcal)	Without grain/cereal (approx. 150 kcal)
1.	1 slice multigrain/whole-wheat toast 1 egg/¼ cup cottage cheese 1 cup milk/buttermilk/vegetable juice 1 cup green tea/tea/coffee without sugar	1 cup milk/yogurt 1 egg/1 cup sprouts 1 tbsp nuts/seeds
2.	⅓ cup high-fibre, sugar-free breakfast cereal/muesli/granola 1 cup milk/yogurt 1 tbsp nuts/seeds	½ cup fruit (cut up) 1 cup milk/yogurt 1 tbsp nuts/seeds
3.	½ cup (cooked) or 2 tbsp (uncooked) oats/finger millet porridge 1 cup milk/yogurt 1 tbsp walnuts/flaxseeds	1 cup fresh fruit and yogurt smoothie* 1 egg/2 tbsp nuts/½ cup sprouts

Options	With grain/cereal (approx. 200 kcal)	Without grain/cereal (approx. 150 kcal)
4.	1 stuffed multigrain chapatti ½ cup yogurt 1 cup green tea/tea/coffee without sugar	¼–½ cup cottage cheese + 1 cup vegetables (sautéed) ½ cup fruit (cut up) 1 cup green tea/tea/coffee without sugar/vegetable juice
5.	½ cup (cooked) or 2 tbsp (uncooked) oats/barley upma + ½ cup vegetables (cut up) 1 cup buttermilk/vegetable juice	1 (medium) besan/moong dal cheela + green chutney 1 cup milk/yogurt/vegetable juice
6.	1 (medium) multigrain pancake 1 cup milk/buttermilk/vegetable juice	1 (medium) besan/moong dal cheela + green chutney 1 cup green tea/tea/coffee without sugar/vegetable juice
7.	¼ cup poha (cooked) + ¼ cup soy granules + ½ cup vegetables (cut up) + 2 tbsp peanuts 1 cup vegetable juice	1 egg/2 egg whites + 1 yolk ½ cup fruit (cut up)
8.	1 missi roti ½ cup yogurt 1 cup green tea/tea/coffee without sugar	1 cup moong dal poha (cooked) + ½ cup vegetables (cut up) 1 cup green tea/tea/coffee without sugar 1 cup vegetable juice

Options	With grain/cereal (approx. 200 kcal)	Without grain/cereal (approx. 150 kcal)
9.	1 triangle/rectangle multigrain sandwich (egg/cheese/cottage cheese/vegetable) 1 cup milk/buttermilk/vegetable juice	½ cup gram (sautéed) + ½ cup vegetables (cut up) 1 cup milk/green tea/tea/coffee without sugar/vegetable juice
10.	2 triangles/rectangles multigrain sandwich (egg/cheese/cottage cheese/vegetable) 1 cup green tea/tea/coffee without sugar	3–4 squares dhokla 1 cup milk/buttermilk/green tea/tea/coffee without sugar/vegetable juice
11.	½ cup quinoa (cooked) + ½ cup vegetables (cut up) + 2 tbsp peanuts 1 cup green tea/tea/coffee without sugar/vegetable juice	1 cup vegetables (sautéed) 1 cup milk/buttermilk/green tea/tea/coffee without sugar/vegetable juice
12.	2 theplas ½ cup yogurt 1 cup green tea/tea/coffee without sugar	2 (medium) tikkis soy/tofu/chana/yogurt/cottage cheese† 1 cup milk/buttermilk/green tea/tea/coffee without sugar/vegetable juice
13.	1 dosa + coconut chutney 1 cup green tea/tea/coffee without sugar/vegetable juice	2 (small) moong dal idlis 1 cup green tea/tea/coffee without sugar/vegetable juice

Notes:

1. Eggs can be cooked as poached, baked, scrambled, fried or as omelettes with less oil in a non-stick pan.
2. Milk and yogurt should be low-fat (<1 per cent), that is, skimmed or double-toned.
3. Vegetable juice should ideally be taken with the pulp. A quarter cup of cut-up fruits may be added.

* For recipe, see p. 168; † For recipe for tofu/cottage cheese tikkis, see p. 173.

Mid-morning snack

A mid-morning snack is needed to evenly distribute your calories to avoid spikes in blood sugar levels and thereby cut cravings. However, if you miss it occasionally, don't fret about it.

For approximately 50–75 kcal:

1. 1–2 tbsp nuts
2. 1 tbsp gram (roasted)
3. ½ cup fruit (cut up)/1 cup coconut water
4. 1 cup lemon water without sugar
5. 1 cup green tea/tea/coffee without sugar

Lunch

For those who are sedentary and need to work at a desk, a big lunch is counterproductive. Use lunch to pack in raw vegetables to keep yourself energized and away from unhealthy snacking. Ensure some protein intake in the form of yogurt, cottage cheese, sprouts, pulses or lean meat to add satiety. If you're going for grains/cereals, choose low-glycaemic options. If your peak-hunger time is evening, treat lunch as a transitory mealtime, having only light foods, and save your grains/cereals for supper.

Table 5.4: The lunch meal plan with options

Options	With grains/ cereals (approx. 350–400 kcal)	Without grains/ cereals (approx. 250–300 kcal)	On-the-go lunch (approx. 150–200 kcal)
1.	1 cup soup/2 cups salad	1 cup soup/2 cups salad	2 cups salad

Options	With grains/ cereals (approx. 350–400 kcal)	Without grains/ cereals (approx. 250–300 kcal)	On-the-go lunch (approx. 150–200 kcal)
	1–2 cups vegetables (cooked)/1–2 cups vegetables (stir-fried) 100–150 gm chicken or fish/¼ cup cottage cheese or tofu/1 cup soy nuggets ½ cup rice (cooked)/½ cup pasta (cooked)/½ cup noodles (cooked)/1 slice multigrain/whole-wheat toast (or as per grain allowance, not exceeding 2 servings of grains/ cereals at any one point)	1–2 cups vegetables (cooked)/1–2 cups vegetables (stir-fried) 100–150 gm chicken or fish/¼ cup cottage cheese or tofu/1 cup soy nuggets	1 cup vegetable juice 1 cup sprouts or 1 cup soy nuggets or ½ cup chickpeas/ rajma/dal or pulse (all boiled) or ½ cup cottage cheese/tofu or 1–2 eggs or 100 gm chicken/ fish
2.	2 cups salad 1–2 cups vegetables (cooked) 1–1½ cups yogurt/ raita 1 chapatti/½ cup rice (cooked)	2 cups salad 1–2 cups vegetables (cooked) 1–1½ cups yogurt/ raita	1 cup milk ½ cup fruit (cut up) 1 cup vegetables (cooked)/1 cup soup

Options	With grains/ cereals (approx. 350–400 kcal)	Without grains/ cereals (approx. 250–300 kcal)	On-the-go lunch (approx. 150–200 kcal)
	(or as per grain allowance, not exceeding 2 servings of grains/cereals at any one point)		
3.	2 cups salad 1–2 cups vegetables (cooked) 1 cup dal/pulse (cooked) 1 chapatti/½ cup rice (cooked) (or as per grain allowance, not exceeding 2 servings of grains/ cereals at any one point)	2 cups salad 1–2 cups vegetables (cooked) 1 cup dal/pulse (cooked)	2 cups salad 1 cup yogurt ½ cup fruit (cut up) ½–1 cup vegetables (cooked)
4.	2 cups salad 1 cup yogurt/raita 1 cup dal 1 chapatti/½ cup rice (or as per grain allowance, not exceeding 2 servings of grains/cereals at any one point)	2 cups salad 1 cup yogurt/raita 1 cup dal	2 cups salad 1 cup sprouts 1 cup yogurt/raita/ buttermilk ½ cup fruit (cut up)

Options	With grains/ cereals (approx. 350–400 kcal)	Without grains/ cereals (approx. 250–300 kcal)	On-the-go lunch (approx. 150–200 kcal)
5.	2 cups salad 1–2 cups sambar Coconut chutney/ tomato chutney 1 (large) or 2 (small) idlis/1 plain dosa/1 (large) or 2 (small) vadas	2 cups salad 1–2 cups sambar 2 (medium) dahi-vada Coconut chutney/ tomato chutney	½ cup fruit (cut up) 1 cup coffee with milk

Notes:

1. Two cups of salad could include 1 carrot, 1 cucumber and 1 tomato.
2. One grain/cereal preparation may be exchanged with another grain/cereal preparation, according to serving sizes, preferences or availability.

Late-afternoon snack

For approximately 50–75 kcal:

1. 1 cup green tea/tea/coffee without sugar
2. 2 tbsp nuts/peanuts/gram/seeds (roasted)
3. ½ cup fruit (cut up)/1 cup coconut water
4. 1 cup lemon water without sugar

Supper: The 7 p.m. meal

This is often the peak-hunger time for most people, especially those who work. If you fall into this category, I would advise you to have a proper meal at this point and have a lighter meal for dinner, which most of us eat much later. In other words, break up your dinner into two meals. Have your grains at this point. However, if you would like to combine the two meals, you must have your dinner by 8 p.m. at the latest; then there will be no conflict. In case you get late, either skip the grain/cereal or go for a short walk.

Table 5.5: The supper meal plan with options

Options	With grains/cereals (approx. 350 kcal)	Without grains/cereals (approx. 200 kcal)
1.	½–1 cup vegetables (cut up or cooked) or ½ cup cottage cheese/tofu or 100 gm chicken 1–2 multigrain chapatti rolls (or as per grain/cereal allowance, not exceeding 2 servings of grains/cereals at any one point)	1–2 cups vegetables (cut up or cooked) 2 besan/moong dal cheelas
2.	1–2 cups vegetables (cut up or cooked) 1–2 chapattis/½ cup rice (cooked) (or as per grain allowance, not exceeding 2 servings of grains/cereals at any one point)	1 cup milk 3–4 (medium) squares dhokla/1 egg/2 egg whites + 1 yolk
3.	1 cup coffee without sugar 2 triangles/rectangles multigrain/whole-wheat sandwich (or as per grain allowance, not exceeding 2 servings of grains/cereals at any one point)	1 cup milk 2 (medium) tikkis tofu/cottage cheese*

Options	With grains/cereals (approx. 350 kcal)	Without grains/cereals (approx. 200 kcal)
4.	1 egg/¼ cup cottage cheese 1–2 slices multigrain/whole-wheat toast (or as per grain allowance, not exceeding 2 servings of grains/cereals at any one point)	1 cup milk ½ cup fruit (cut up) 1–2 tbsp nuts/peanuts
5.	1 cup green tea/tea/coffee without sugar 2 cups multigrain bhel (1 cup puffed rice + 1 cup vegetables [cut up] + 2 tbsp peanuts)	1 fresh fruit and yogurt smoothie† 1 tbsp nuts/peanuts/ gram (roasted)
6.	1–2 cups vegetables (cut up or cooked) ½–1 cup pasta (cooked)/2–4 slices pizza (thin crust) (or as per grain allowance, not exceeding 2 servings of grains/cereals at any one point)	1 cup milk 2 soy cutlets‡

Note: One grain/cereal preparation may be exchanged with another grain/cereal preparation, according to serving sizes, preferences or availability.
* For recipe, see p. 173; † For recipe, see p. 168; ‡ For recipe, see p. 171.

Dinner

We tend to eat dinner late and, as I've said, one of the most important things about keeping your weight down is to have a light meal when it's late. I would recommend avoiding grain/cereal intake during this meal, particularly for those who have metabolic obesity or insulin resistance.

Table 5.6: The dinner meal plan with options

Options	With grains/cereals (approx. 300 kcal)	Without grains/cereals (approx. 150–200 kcal)
1.	1–2 cups vegetables (cooked)/soup/salad 100–150 gm chicken/fish ½ cup rice (cooked)/½ cup pasta (cooked)/½ cup noodles (cooked)/1 slice multigrain/whole-wheat toast (or as per grain allowance, not exceeding 2 servings of grains/cereals at any one point)	1–2 cups vegetables (cooked)/soup/salad
2.	1 cup soup/salad 1–2 cups vegetables (cooked) ¼ cup cottage cheese or tofu/1 cup soy nuggets ½ cup rice (cooked)/½ cup pasta (cooked)/½ cup noodles (cooked)/1 slice multigrain/whole-wheat toast (or as per grain allowance, not exceeding 2 servings of grains/cereals at any one point)	1 cup soup/salad 1–2 cups vegetables (cooked) 100–150 gm chicken or fish ¼ cup cottage cheese or tofu/1 cup soy nuggets
3.	2 cups salad 1–2 cups vegetables (cooked) 1–1½ cups yogurt/raita/1 cup dal (cooked) 1 chapatti/½ cup rice (cooked)	1–2 cups vegetables (cut up or cooked) 1–1½ cups yogurt/raita

Options	With grains/cereals (approx. 300 kcal)	Without grains/cereals (approx. 150–200 kcal)
4.	2 cups salad/1 cup soup 1–2 cups soup/salad 1–2 cups vegetables (stir-fried) + ½ cup rice (cooked)/½ cup pasta (cooked)/½ cup spaghetti (cooked)	1–2 cups vegetables (cooked) 1 cup dal (cooked)
5.	2 cups salad 1–2 cups sambar 2 (small) idlis	1 cup milk/yogurt/green tea ½ cup fruit (cut up) 2 tbsp nuts

Notes: One grain/cereal preparation may be exchanged with another grain/cereal preparation, according to serving sizes, preferences or availability.

Post-dinner snack

For approximately 50 kcal:

1. 1 cup green tea/tea/coffee without sugar/½ cup milk
2. 1–2 tbsp nuts/2 tbsp gram (roasted)/½ cup fruit (cut up)

Supplements

During a weight-loss programme, a judicious use of supplements is recommended, under the supervision of a qualified practitioner.

Sample meal plan

Table 5.7: Sample meal plan for 1200 kcal (3-grain/cereal allowance)

Meals	Menu
Breakfast	1 cup milk/yogurt ¼ cup high-fibre, sugar-free breakfast cereal (muesli/granola) 1 tbsp nuts/seeds
Mid-morning snack	1 cup green tea/tea/coffee without sugar ½ cup fruit (cut up)
Lunch	2 cups salad 1–2 cups vegetables (cooked) 1–1½ cups yogurt or raita/1 cup sprouts
Late-afternoon snack	1 cup green tea/tea/coffee without sugar 1–2 tbsp peanuts/2 tbsp gram (roasted)
Supper Option 1	1–2 multigrain chapatti roll (vegetables/ cottage cheese/chicken) (or as per grain allowance, not exceeding 2 servings of grains/cereals at any one point)
Option 2	2 triangles/rectangles multigrain/whole-wheat sandwich (toasted or untoasted) (or as per grain allowance, not exceeding 2 servings of grains/cereals at any one point)

Meals	Menu
Dinner	1 cup soup/salad 1–2 cups vegetables (cooked) 100–150 gm chicken or fish/¼ cup cottage cheese/1 cup dal (cooked)
Post-dinner snack	1 cup green tea/tea/coffee without sugar 1–2 tbsp nuts

Special menus

Over the year there are certain phases when it becomes difficult to maintain your diet. Here are some meal plans that might come in handy.

During fasts

During fasts, plan one major meal with alternative grains, prepared in less fat, to be had ideally before sunset. Snack on milk, yogurt, fruits, nuts, seeds and dry fruits—and you have a diet that can help you drop those kilos and boost energy!

A sound fasting programme must ensure the following:

1. Eat less but not starve.
2. Include plenty of fluids, water, fresh fruits and vegetables.
3. Include foods rich in micronutrients, antioxidants and phytochemicals.
4. Include variety through alternative foods and ensure good nutrition.
5. Break your fast with coconut water/milk/yogurt/buttermilk/vegetable or fruit juice/soup/fruits.

6. Keep your stomach light and do not eat too much immediately after breaking a fast.

These principles conform to scientific principles of nutrition.

During Navaratras, alternative grains are eaten and traditional staples like wheat, rice, pulses and most vegetables are prohibited. Even those who do not observe fasts often avoid eggs, fish, poultry and meat, and some even stop eating garlic and onions. Many avoid alcohol during this period.

Sample meal plan for fasts

Table 5.8: Sample meal plan for fasts

Meals	Regular fasts	Navaratra fasts
Breakfast	1 cup milk ½ cup fruit (cut up) 4 almonds + 1 walnut + 2 raisins	1 cup milk ½ cup fruit (cut up) 4 almonds + 1 walnut + 2 raisins
Mid-morning snack	1 cup vegetable juice/ coconut water	1 cup green tea/tea/coffee without sugar/buttermilk
Lunch Option 1	1–1½ cups yogurt ½ cup fruit (cut up)	1–1½ cups yogurt ½ cup fruit (cut up)
Option 2	2 cups salad 1 cup sprouts	2 cups salad ¼ cup cottage cheese/tofu
Late-afternoon snack Option 1	1 cup green tea/tea/coffee without sugar 2–3 tbsp peanuts	1–2 cups vegetables (cooked) 1–2 chapattis (buckwheat/ chestnut/amaranth)

Meals	Regular fasts	Navaratra fasts
Option 2	½–1 cup yogurt/raita 1–2 tbsp seeds (watermelon seeds/ melon seeds/lotus seeds/ sunflower seeds/flaxseeds)	½–1 cup yogurt/raita ½–1 cup high-fibre rice (samak chawal); (cooked)/ sago khichri with peanuts
Evening snack	1 cup soup	1 cup green tea/tea/coffee without sugar/coconut water 1–2 tbsp seeds (watermelon seeds/melon seeds/lotus seeds/sunflower seeds/ flaxseeds)
Dinner Option 1	1 cup milk ½ cup fruit (cut up)	1–1½ cups yogurt ½ cup fruit (cut up) 1–2 cups vegetables (cooked)/1 cup soup or cottage cheese salad
Option 2	1 fresh fruit smoothie	1 cup fresh fruit smoothie 2 tbsp nuts

On the fast track: The rapid weight-loss plan

I am not a believer of the quick-fix weight-loss plan as you know but some of you may well need to lose weight fast for a specific event. If you must, then follow the meal plan outlined in Table 5.9, p. 122. On an average, the diet should be between 600 and 800 kcal and the expected weight loss not more than 5–6 kg in 2 weeks. However, you must remember that the success of VLCDs can be rather short-lived because water and muscle are lost from the body, rather than excess body fat. Once normal eating is resumed, body fluids are quickly replaced and there is an immediate weight gain. Fasting with juices and water can also be a risky practice, and extreme diets are quite precarious for people with established health issues like diabetes, kidney disease and heart problems.

Those on a fast-track diet must ensure the following:

1. Have a nutritionally balanced diet under the supervision of a qualified professional.
2. Don't over-restrict or binge.
3. Include plenty of fluids
4. Exercise for at least 1 hour every day.
5. Follow up with a maintenance plan and behaviour modification.

For a sample diet plan for rapid weight loss, see Table 5.9, p. 122.

Table 5.9: The rapid weight-loss diet plan

Meal	Day 1	Day 2	Day 3	Day 4	Day 5	Day 6	Day 7
Early-morning snack	1 cup green tea/tea/coffee without sugar 7 almonds	1 cup green tea/tea/coffee without sugar 3 walnuts	1 cup green tea/tea/coffee without sugar 7 pistachios	1 cup green tea/tea/coffee without sugar 1 tbsp sunflower seeds	1 cup green tea/tea/coffee without sugar 5 cashews	1 cup green tea/tea/coffee without sugar 1 tbsp pumpkin seeds	1 cup green tea/tea/coffee without sugar 7 almonds
Breakfast	1 egg/½ cup cottage cheese ½ cup seasonal fruit (cut up) 1 cup green tea/tea/coffee without sugar	½ cup tofu ½ cup seasonal fruit (cut up) 1 cup green tea/tea/coffee without sugar	1 cup moong sprouts 1 cup buttermilk 1 cup green tea/tea/coffee without sugar	1 cheela 1 cup chhaach 1 cup green tea/tea/coffee without sugar	1 cup milk ½ cup seasonal fruit (cut up) 1 cup green tea/tea/coffee without sugar	½ cup yogurt 1 tbsp walnut (crushed) ¼ cup apple (cut up) 1 cup green tea/tea/coffee without sugar	1 egg/½ cup cottage cheese 1 slice multigrain/whole-wheat toast 1 cup green tea/tea/coffee without sugar

Meal	Day 1	Day 2	Day 3	Day 4	Day 5	Day 6	Day 7
Mid-morning snack	1 cup lemon water without sugar	1 cup amla water without sugar	1 cup vegetable juice without sugar	1 cup coconut water	1 cup jamun juice without sugar	1 cup grapefruit juice/ buttermilk without sugar	1 cup coconut water
Lunch	1 cup salad ⅓ cup gram (cooked)/dal (cooked)/ rajma (cooked) 1 cup seasonal vegetables (cut up)	1 cup yogurt/ raita 1 cup seasonal vegetables (cut up)	1 cup soup 1–2 cups salad	1 cup yogurt or raita ½ cup fruit (cut up)	2 cups salad 1 cup seasonal vegetables (cooked)	1 cup yogurt/ raita 1 cup seasonal vegetables (cooked)	1 cup soup 1–2 cups salad

Meals	Day 1	Day 2	Day 3	Day 4	Day 5	Day 6	Day 7
Evening snack	1 cup green tea/tea/coffee without sugar ½ cup snacks (roasted)	1 cup green tea/tea/coffee without sugar ½ cup snacks (roasted)	1 cup green tea/tea/coffee without sugar ½ cup snacks (roasted)	1 cup green tea/tea/coffee without sugar ½ cup snacks (roasted)	1 cup green tea/tea/coffee without sugar 100–150 gm chicken or fish/½ cup cottage cheese or tofu/1 cup soy	1 cup green tea/tea/coffee without sugar 100–150 gm chicken or fish/½ cup cottage cheese or tofu/1 cup soy	1 cup green tea/tea/coffee without sugar 100–150 gm chicken or fish/½ cup cottage cheese or tofu/1 cup soy
Dinner	1 cup soup or double-toned/skimmed milk Fibre supplement						

Note: You may have an unlimited amount of 'free' foods—green tea without sugar/tea without sugar/coffee without sugar/clear soups/green salad, etc.

Sample meal plan for metabolic obesity/insulin resistance/PCOS

The meal plan for PCOS must focus on small, frequent meals, limiting grain/cereal and fruit intake and including nuts, seeds, adequate protein and low-fat dairy.

Table 5.10: Sample meal plan for metabolic obesity/insulin resistance/PCOS (2-grain/cereal allowance)

Meals	Menu
Early-morning snack	1 cup green tea without sugar 1 cup lemon/amla water without sugar
Breakfast Option 1	1 cup milk 2 tbsp muesli/2 tbsp oats or barley (uncooked)
Option 2	1 egg/¼ cup cottage cheese 1 slice multigrain/whole-wheat toast
Option 3	1 cup cold coffee without sugar 1 (medium) cheela
Option 4	1 cup vegetable juice 1 cup sprouts/1 egg/2 whites + 1 yolk/¼ cup cottage cheese
Mid-morning snack	1 cup lemon water/green tea/tea/coffee without sugar 1 tbsp nuts
Lunch	2 cups salad 1–2 cups vegetables (cooked) or 1–1½ cups yogurt/raita or 1 cup sprouts or 1 cup dal (cooked)

Meals	Menu
Late-afternoon snack	1 cup green tea/tea/coffee without sugar ½ cup fruit (cut up) 1–2 tbsp nuts/peanuts/gram (roasted)
Supper Option 1	1 cup green tea/tea/coffee without sugar 1– 1½ cups multigrain bhel
Dinner	1–2 cups salad/1 cup soup/1–2 cups vegetables (cooked) 100–150 gm chicken or fish/½ cup cottage cheese or tofu
Post-dinner snack	1 cup green tea/tea/coffee without sugar

Things to remember:

1. Avoid potatoes, colocasia, mangoes, bananas and fruit juices.
2. Limit the intake of melons and watermelons.
3. The following are safe to include:
   a. Low-fat dairy.
   b. 2–3 tbsp gram (roasted)/½ cup namkeen (roasted).
   c. 1–2 tbsp peanuts/nuts/seeds.
4. Preferred sweets include raisins or figs or peanut or sesame balls/1–2 tbsp honey-coated almonds/1–2 cubes dark chocolate.

✚ ADDING IT ALL UP

If you are aware of your required caloric intake, start by making a note of how many servings of each food group you require in a day. If not, proceed to the diet plans and recommendations, and plan your diet accordingly. If I had to summarize, I would simply say: use the half-plate rule, minimize sugars, reduce the grains/cereals to half and fill up on vegetables. Also include at least 2–3 servings of good protein through pulses, low-fat dairy, lean meats and fats through nuts and seeds.

6

MANAGING THE PROBLEM AREAS

✚ THE DOCTOR SAYS

In the previous chapter I gave you detailed options on how to regulate your eating. But what happens when you aren't at home? The problem with diets is that for most of us they work only when we can actively control our food. But let's face it—we are not at home for most of the day. Either we are in college, school or at work; even at home there are those special occasions like celebrations and festivals, when our diet regimens are likely to get thrown off track. I have put together a list of most of these high-risk times, and have come up with solutions to suit each environment. A good diet plan is one which is flexible and one you can improvise as you go ahead so that healthy eating can be a long-term affair. I really do believe that once you internalize the different food groups and the servings of foods you may have from each group daily, along with the principles of healthy eating, you will almost master the art of eating right and will be able to manage your diet routine, whether you're eating out or during those special occasions, no matter what part of the world you are in.

Eating out

Most of us enjoy eating out and today going to a restaurant is a regular occurrence. Many of my clients eat out frequently, twice a week on an average, while in the past going out was considered a real treat. If you are a regular restaurant goer, you need to discipline yourself when you go out as it takes a toll on your weight.

The biggest problem areas when eating out are as follows:

1. Increased temptation.
2. Larger portions.
3. Higher intake of refined starches (maida, cornflour), poor-quality fat, sugar and salt.

With a little effort, eating out can be a joyful experience without it conflicting with your weight-loss goals. Here are a few tips you could try, when eating out:

1. Plan your day in advance.
2. In general, when eating and drinking out, plan ahead and decide how much you would like to eat or drink—and stick to it. Don't just drift into an evening of eating and drinking without thought. Anticipate social pressure and also prepare yourself to deal with it.
3. In a restaurant, avoid buffets; go ala carte.
4. If you have to eat buffet, take a look at all the food that is there, step back and then decide what really tempts you. **Take one helping and remember your portions and the half-plate rule.**
5. Before going to a restaurant, drink one or two glasses of water or eat a piece of fruit to curb your appetite. When you go to a party, eating a light home-cooked meal or snack like vegetables, yogurt, nuts, seeds, dal or salad can be useful.
6. Start your meals with appetizers like clear soups or salads. When unsure about hygiene, avoid uncooked salads and raw preparations.
7. Share the main course or order soups and salads or appetizers instead of main meals. Ask for the salad dressings on the side.

8. If you like variety and want to try different things, order a variety of starters (preferably non-fried), rather than a heavy main course.
9. Skip the breadbasket. While waiting, ask for olives or vegetable sticks.
10. Look for grilled and roasted preparations. Avoid dishes that require too much frying. Pick lean cuts of meat.
11. Go for the vegetables. Ask for the fries and potatoes to be replaced with vegetables. One must look for vegetables with less gravy or without gravy as gravies are loaded with fat and calories. Try grilled vegetables with olive oil.
12. Choose oriental/Mediterranean cuisine over cuisines offering oily gravies.
13. Avoid large meals, particularly late at night.
14. Limit the intake of alcoholic beverages—avoid drinking more than 1–2 medium glasses of wine or other alcoholic beverages before the meal. Alcohol fuels the appetite and reduces awareness. Calories from alcohol are stored preferentially as fats.
15. Snack smart—go for roasted or low-calorie snacks. Remember to order snacks which provide few calories in large portions.
16. Do not be afraid to ask for your foods to be prepared without high-fat ingredients or sauces.
17. Skip desserts if possible, or choose fruits, fruit-based sorbets, tea or coffee. If temptation takes over you, take care to avoid creamy and deep-fried desserts, or share your favourite ones with your friends.
18. Eat less or reduce your portion sizes.
19. Balance out your diet through the day—if you've had a heavy meal, make sure the subsequent meal is light.
20. Stay clear of desserts or foods you do not wish to eat. The sight and smell of food can entice you.

Tips for north Indian dining

1. Choose tandoori food.
2. Avoid curried items; if you find that you can't, then be sure to take out the pieces from the curry. The gravy has the most fat.
3. Go for dry vegetable preparations instead of rich gravies.
4. Avoid dishes like dal makhani and other preparations with cream. If you can't, ask for your order to be made without cream or ladle your serving from the bottom of the vessel as most of the fat lies on the top. As a rule, take smaller portions—a fraction of what you normally would.
5. Avoid parathas, puris and pulao. Go in for ungreased chapattis or steamed rice. Half a cup rice (cooked) = 1 serving of grains/cereals. (See section on grains/cereals, p. 56.)
6. Whole-wheat tandoori roti is preferable to breads made of refined flour like naans, puris, parathas, etc.
7. If your grain/cereal allowance is over for the day, use yogurt, salad or fruits as substitutes.
8. Don't forget that chaat is a masked form of fried foods. If you can't avoid it, do account for the calories. Reduce papris or have non-fried/baked ones.
9. Avoid khoya-based and deep-fried desserts.

Tips for south Indian dining

1. This cuisine is essentially grain/cereal based, with rice-, rawa- or dal-based preparations.
2. Idlis and dosas are high–glycaemic index foods. Try and keep them within your grain/cereal allowance. One (large) idli or

½ (large) dosa without masala or 1 (medium) plain dosa = 1 grain/cereal allowance. (See section on grains/cereals, p. 56.)

3. Avoid potato-based masalas in dosas and go for dal-based dosas, if there is an option in the menu.
4. Dal vadas, well squeezed and drained on tissue, also make a good choice.
5. Dahi-vadas with rasam, and sambar with vegetables are good fillers.
6. Remember, high-starch foods, when eaten late in the evening, may be a problem, especially for those with insulin resistance, and may lead to water retention for those who are carbohydrate or salt sensitive.
7. For non-vegetarians, chicken, fish or prawns with vegetables along with a measured portion of grains/cereals is a good idea.
8. Keep away from heavy gravies and desserts.

Tips for Chinese dining

1. Start the meal with a large helping of soup, preferably without thickening—avoid sweetcorn-, noodle- and wonton-based soups.
2. Go easy on fried appetizers. If the dim sum has been prepared with thick skins, peel some of them off.
3. Order steamed rice instead of fried rice. Portion the rice or noodles according to your grain/cereal allowance.
4. Remember the half-plate rule. Fill up at least half your plate with vegetables.
5. Lightly stir-fried vegetables, tofu, chicken or fish are good choices.
6. Steamed fish with vegetables is hugely satisfying and ticks all the boxes.

7. Be aware that meat and poultry in sweet-and-sour dishes is typically batter coated and deep-fried.
8. Ask for your meal to be made without 'MSG', which is very high in sodium.

Tips for Italian dining

1. Skip bread and breadsticks. Ask for olives or a salad instead.
2. Choose grilled seafood, lean meats or breast of chicken with vegetables.
3. Ask for more vegetables in your pasta. Half a cup pasta (cooked) = 1 serving of grains/cereals. (See section on grains/cereals, p. 56.)
4. Choose thin-crust pizzas over the regular ones. Two slices of thin-crust pizza = 1 serving of grains/cereals.
5. White cream, Alfredo and Marsala sauces tend to be high in fat and calories unless the recipe has been modified. Try a tomato-based sauce instead.
6. Add a dash of Parmesan cheese or olive oil to dishes—they add to the taste and make you feel satiated.

Tips for Greek/Lebanese dining

1. Go for falafel, chicken kebabs or fish with salad.
2. Restrict pittas and wraps as per your grain/cereal allowance. (See section on grains/cereals, p. 56.)
3. Avoid heavy desserts like baklava.

Tips for Mexican dining

1. Order sour cream and guacamole on the side, and pile up on the salsa, which is naturally low in fat, instead.
2. Order soft tacos rather than crispy, fried ones.
3. If you order a taco salad, go easy on the deep-fried shell.
4. Go easy on nachos and cheese. Order a low-fat appetizer such as tortilla soup or gazpacho instead.
5. Choose a regular entrée instead of a combination platter, which may be high in fat and calories.
6. Keep your grain/cereal allowance in mind. Good choices include rice and beans, tamales, tostadas, and enchildas stuffed with vegetables, shrimp or chicken.

Occupational vulnerabilities

Our jobs tend to define our eating habits. Office jobs take up at least 8 hours of the day, and you need to secure this environment when it comes to your diet and fitness. With sedentary jobs the risks only increase. Here's a list of common situations where you might find it difficult to stick to your diet regimen, along with tips and solutions that can help you keep your diet on track.

The corporate executive/office worker

1. Try to eat regular meals. Your day should begin with breakfast, followed by a mid-morning snack, lunch, an early-evening snack and then dinner (which should be had as early as possible). Plan your meals as per the meal plans given in Chapter 5. Small meals

with light snacks work better. Avoid long gaps between meals as well as skipping meals.

2. As far as possible eat a light lunch. Go for a salad, soup, sprouts, beans, lean meats, nuts, yogurt and fruit lunch. Grain-/cereal-free meals will keep you more energized.
3. Choose to have home-made food on a day-to-day basis. Avoid office cafeterias; when this is not possible, follow the tips for dining out given earlier in this chapter (p. 131).
4. Snack smart. Snacking is one of the biggest problem areas for anyone working in an office. One way to control this is to bring your own snack box to the office. Sprouts, popcorn, fresh fruits, nuts and seeds, raisins and other dried fruits, yogurt, roasted whole grains, and whole-wheat bread sandwiches are all good options. Cereals make for an excellent early-evening snack. Evening is certainly the time when hunger strikes the hardest and self-control is at its weakest. Make the evening a mealtime. Fruits, nuts, seeds and dried fruits are good as mid-morning snacks.
5. For those who work until late, breaking up the meals and dividing calories between office and home will help prevent the loading up of calories late at night. Consume grains/cereals before 8 p.m. and reserve vegetables, pulses, milk or fruits for later.
6. Limit or avoid sugar-laden beverages. Nimbu-pani, sugar-free aam panna, iced tea without sugar, fruit-based, sugar-free beverages and lassi are some of the healthier options.
7. If you are obliged to have tea/coffee frequently during meetings, go for green tea, decaffeinated coffee or herbal teas like camomile, jasmine, etc. Limit the quantity of tea/coffee to half a cup and watch the sugar you take with it.

8. Make time for exercise.
   a. Find opportunities to take short, brisk walks within your office complex intermittently during the day. This will energize you as you burn calories.
   b. Aim to exercise regularly for 60 minutes on most days of the week.
   c. Brisk walking, swimming, jogging, dancing and cycling are some examples of good exercise.
9. Manage stress. Stress and emotions can make you eat mindlessly. Eat only when hungry. Learn the difference between physiological and psychological hunger. Some practical tips to manage stress are given below:
   a. Avoid overeating when fatigued or too stressed.
   b. Be optimistic.
   c. Practise time management.
   d. Avoid excessive caffeine, alcohol and tobacco.
   e. Try and get 6–8 hours of sleep daily.
   f. Spend at least 1 hour a day with family.
   g. Take regular breaks. Try to holiday every 3 months with family.
   h. Listening to relaxing music is therapeutic and calming.
   i. Consider having a pet. Stroking an animal has been found to be relaxing.
   j. Learn to recognize your own threshold for stress and do not push yourself past it.

Travel, meetings and conferences

These can really throw you off your diet and exercise regimen.

1. Plan your day and reserve most of your food intake for social engagements.
2. Avoid heavy dinners. If unavoidable, then skip the grains/cereals and sweets.
3. Balance out your diet the next day.
4. Eat healthy during meetings and avoid unnecessary snacking on biscuits or fried foods.
5. If possible, keep lunch light.
6. Watch your alcohol intake.
7. Conferences offer buffets with rich food. Follow the principles of dining out given earlier in this chapter (p. 131).
8. When travelling, ensure you carry healthy snacks like nuts and fruits, so you do not need to snack on unhealthy foods at airports, etc.
9. Try and stick to your exercise regimen as far as possible.

Holidays

Vacations are meant to recharge you. However, how you treat yourself on a vacation determines whether this is what happens. More often than not, people overindulge in food and drink and go off their exercise schedules; not only does this make people gain weight but it also makes them feel sluggish and tired.

1. Be active. If you exercise regularly, don't stop. Continue to exercise during your holiday. Check if the hotel you've booked has a gym,

or else go for walks, run, swim, play sports or cycle outdoors.

2. Choose one favourite meal for the day and plan other meals accordingly. The other meals could be light, consisting of salads, vegetables and soups. Breakfast buffets can throw you off, so plan to eat appropriately.
3. If possible, schedule holiday dinners at normal mealtimes. Having meals outside of normal mealtimes, particularly late-night large meals, contributes to overeating. Lavish meals in succession can be balanced out by keeping a few meals very light, with milk, fruits, soups, salads, etc.
4. Carry appropriate snack foods like seeds, roasted nuts or whole grains to munch on, so you are not forced to buy unhealthy snacks off the shelf.
5. Watch your drinks. Count your alcohol calories and include these under your grain/cereal allowance.
6. Towards the end of your holiday, make a few dinners light. It'll help you balance out the excesses.

Manage your sweet cravings the right way

Most of us enjoy sweets and desserts. Some, however, have a compulsive sweet tooth. Sugar can get addictive—the more you have the more you want—so trying to manage those cravings is worthwhile. You have to break out of the vicious cycle.

1. Limit refined carbohydrates. Carbohydrate-rich foods like white breads, pastas and so forth might not taste sweet, but they are forms of sugar. Choose healthy and low–glycaemic index

carbohydrates instead, like whole grains, barley, oats, pulses, fruits rich in fibre, and vegetables.

2. Sugar cravings are often a consequence of missing nutrients. These include proteins, good fats, B vitamins, magnesium, chromium and zinc. So a handful of nuts, seeds or roasted gram might be a good thing to reach for when you are craving that chocolate cake.

Table 6.1: Sources of nutrients

Nutrients	Sources
Proteins	Pulses, soybean, tofu, egg, chicken, fish and lean meats, nuts and seeds
Essential fats	Cold-pressed oils, nuts, seeds, fatty fish and seafood
B vitamins	Fresh fruits, vegetables, whole grains, nuts, seeds, dairy and pulses
Zinc	Seafood, meat, poultry, whole grains, nuts and seeds

3. Fresh fruits and dry fruits like raisins, apricots, figs, dates, etc. should be your preferred sweets.
4. 'Sugar-free' fixes include mouth fresheners like fennel, cardamom and sugar-free gums. Avoid these.
5. Keep healthier snack options such as dark chocolate, and honey-coated, jaggery-coated and chocolate-coated nuts.
6. Increase the intake of raw vegetables.
7. Drinking lemon water, unsweetened tea/coffee, hot chocolate or a little sugar-sweetened tea/coffee also helps control sugar craving. If you are prone to sugar lows, make sure you eat something at regular intervals.

8. Try and assess how often you have sugar cravings during the day. If you find yourself giving in to them frequently, set yourself a target—that you will fight them more than giving in to them.
9. Be conscious and aware whenever you have these cravings.
10. Lose belly fat.
11. Exercise regularly.

7

FIFTEEN PRINCIPLES OF EATING: A SUMMARY

✚ THE DOCTOR SAYS

Weaving the information you have gained from this book with the principles of healthy eating, regular exercise and common sense will help you get in shape in the most healthy and realistic way possible. In this chapter I want to move beyond meal plans and the science and look at our long-term goals. You can lose all your weight following my diet plans—but you need to keep it off too. This is in fact harder than losing weight and is a rather neglected area. Inculcating healthy and mindful eating habits for life is key. Here are fifteen principles for keeping the weight off for good.

1. Keep up your motivation

When ready to give up on your diet, remember this—the difference between a successful person and an unsuccessful person is that the successful person never stops trying.

a. Don't blame your genes. Even if your genes have a propensity for obesity and diabetes, you have no excuse for being overweight or obese. It just means that you have to work harder and walk a tighter rope than others. Making and sticking with lifestyle changes can help everyone.
b. Stop making excuses and assume full responsibility for your weight.
c. Make yourself feel important. Focus on yourself without feeling guilty. You are worth it!

d. Nothing succeeds like success—reward success. Don't wait to reach your final goal. Get yourself a new dress or a health cookbook or simply indulge in retail therapy.
e. Develop negative associations with undesirable foods and being fat.
f. Develop a positive association with the kind of clothes that you would love to wear. Don't buy larger sizes; rather try to get into your old clothes.
g. When faced with temptation, talk to yourself; think of all the hard work and effort that went into losing that weight and ask yourself: 'How will I feel tomorrow if I don't eat this food today?' Give yourself permission to eat if feelings of deprivation arise.
h. Divert your mind from food by being busy or away from home, talking to your friends or going out.
i. Do not succumb to fad or novel diets. Nutrition quackery is rampant and this is largely an unregulated sector with plenty of self-styled practitioners.
j. When seeking professional advice, carry out thorough research and background checks on the experts you are considering. Do not hesitate to ask questions; it's your right as a client.

2. Set goals

a. Set reasonable and realistic goals. Have short-term and long-term goals.
b. Achieve your ideal BMI and aim for a flat belly. Follow a healthy diet and exercise regularly to achieve an ideal BMI—that is, less than 23 kg per m². The ideal waist circumference is less than

80 cm (approximately 31.5 inches) for women and less than 90 cm (approximately 35.5 inches) for men.

c. Picture the effect weight loss will have on you, how different your life will be and what you would be able to do differently.

d. Think of a strategy that will help you attain that goal.
   1. Make a diet plan for yourself and stick to it.
   2. Exercise regularly for at least 60 minutes 6 days a week.
   3. Keep up your motivation and resist the temptation to eat unhealthy foods.
   4. Write your goals down and put them up where you can see them every day.

e. Buy yourself a good digital weighing scale, better still the kind that gives your body composition analysis as well.

f. Weigh yourself as often as you wish. There are no rules any more. Compare readings weekly.

3. Plan your eating regimen

a. Plan your meals and snacks in advance. Snack smart.

b. Most social activities revolve around food, so plan your day accordingly.

c. Start your day with breakfast, even if it is a light one. People who eat breakfast take in fewer calories throughout the remainder of the day. Choose a low–glycaemic index breakfast. Studies have shown that people who eat small meals through the day are able to control their appetite well.

d. Make sure your dinner time falls between 6.30 and 8 p.m. If you find that it is getting late, keep your dinner light.

e. Eat your favourite food once a week.
f. Keep indulgence to no more than one meal a week and do not go overboard.
g. Watch your weekend indulgence. Often, people who do very well through the week allow themselves to relax over the weekend, which leads to weight gain on Monday morning. Following the diet regimen during the week brings down the weight by the weekend only for it to go up the following Monday. This keeps them from losing weight, much to their amazement.
h. Make diet changes that can be maintained for life; quick fixes are counterproductive for healthy weight management.
i. Travel smart. (See section on travel, meetings and conferences, p. 140.)
j. Follow your diet during holidays. (See section on holidays, p. 140.)
k. Create a timeline. You've started making those small changes already. What is your plan for the next week? What do you need to do to reach from point A (your last weigh-in) to point B (your next weigh-in)?
l. Don't let lapses become collapses—have a contingency plan. Parties, weddings, eating out, etc. will always happen. Plan ahead. If you know you're going somewhere where you may eat more, make the previous meal really light. If it's an unexpected outing, balance your meals out the next day.
m. Track your progress. Make sure the results you are hoping to achieve are measurable—for example, 'I want to lose 1 kg in a week'. Focus more on short-term/weekly goals, and measure your progress. Don't get overwhelmed by the 'big picture'—that you have to lose these many kilos in all.

n. Reward yourself from time to time in a reasonable and smart way—not through a 'chocathon' on the weekend, for example.

4. Practise mindful eating

a. Maintain a food diary.
b. Increase your awareness.
c. Learn the difference between psychological and physiological hunger.
d. Pay attention to what you choose rather than what you forgo. Don't fool yourself by focusing on all the food that you did not eat and feel sorry for yourself. You may be still overloading on calories, even if you didn't touch most of that buffet!
e. Focus on your food. Enjoy how it looks and tastes and notice how much you're eating.
f. Eat slowly, chew thoroughly and take smaller bites. What's the rush? Savour the food. You will enjoy it more and eat less.
g. Pre-plate your food, so that you can see exactly what you are eating. Mostly, people tend to eat less if they put everything on their plate in one go, like in the case of a traditional thali or the Japanese bento box, and are able to see how much they are going to eat. However, if you like to keep busy with food for longer, you may go for seconds and thirds as long as you keep the portions small.
h. Postpone that second helping by 20 minutes—the time it usually takes for you to realize you don't need it. It takes that much time for the stomach to send the signal indicating that it is full to the brain.
i. Consult your nutritionist and know appropriate portion sizes and

calorie content of foods.

j. Practise portion control:
    1. Use smaller plates and bowls.
    2. Make smaller-sized idlis, cutlets, tikkis, chapattis, etc. We subconsciously treat numbers as a yardstick to judge how much we have eaten. For example, we tend to feel more satiated if we have 2 small chapattis than when we have 1 big/medium chapatti.

k. Remember the principles of healthy eating—context, variety, balance and moderation. (See section on the principles of healthy eating, p. 98.)

l. Do not let food be too accessible, especially at work, if you are a compulsive eater. Seek professional help if needed.

m. Identify your cravings and discuss them with your nutritionist.

n. Do not compare yourself to others. Remember, you are unique.

o. Pay attention to how you are feeling. Your moods can affect your food intake. People often eat when they are feeling tired, angry, upset or bored. Find the proper activity to deal with the specific feeling—eating is not it! If you are tired, take a catnap or go for a walk; if you are angry, talk to a friend or do something you love to do; if you are bored, make a phone call to someone you have not spoken with for a long time or make a list of all the things you have put off doing for some reason. Choose one thing from the list and start doing it. Learn to cope with emotional eating and boredom.

p. Don't let family eating patterns disrupt your dietary discipline.

q. Keep your home stocked with fruits and vegetables.

r. Avoid eating while watching television or reading.

s. Sip water between bites. It will slow you down.

t. Eat small, frequent meals. Avoid eating large meals, particularly at night, as they promote weight gain.
u. Do not skip meals.
v. Do not starve yourself.
w. Don't fall for the 'don't waste' dictum. Do not scavenge for leftovers. To deal with your perceived need to 'clean your plate', remember that excess food goes either to waste or to the waist.

5. Be food wise

a. Train your palate. Eating healthy and increasing your intake of raw vegetables and vegetable juices substantially can help you train your palate. You will realize that you have lost the taste for unhealthy food.
b. Try out different cuisines.
c. Make losing weight enjoyable. Eat something that you like once a day, ideally at your peak-hunger time.
d. Avoid grains/cereals at the beginning of the meal; if you don't, chances are you will end up eating too large a quantity. Start with soup, salad and vegetables, and shift the grains/cereals to the end of the meal. This will help you limit their intake and stay within your grain/cereal allowance.
e. Choose healthy sweets. If possible, replace sweets with fruits.
f. Ensure adequate protein intake.
g. Eat fresh fruits and fresh or steamed vegetables for satiety. Ensure adequate fibre intake.
h. Increase fluid/water intake through the day; thirst should not be mistaken for hunger.
i. Choose healthy, low-calorie beverages.

j. Late-night fixes may include dark chocolate, hot chocolate (preferably without sugar), roasted gram, seeds, nuts or some fruits. Never load up late at night.
k. Increase the levels of phytochemicals through fruits and vegetables, as diets rich in these favour weight loss.
l. Keep a check on alcohol and smoking. If trying to quit, avoid the company of those who drink or smoke too much.
m. Cook interesting food/cuisines. Invest in cookbooks. Use different ingredients and sauces as you are expected to change the way you eat on a long-term basis. (See recipes in Chapter 8, p. 159) You must look forward to your meals.
n. Make interesting low-fat dips and fruit salads. Try out new soups. Present your food attractively.
o. Keep a healthy kitchen. Switch to healthier cookware and methods of cooking. Use pans, pressure cookers, slow cookers, steamers, oil sprays and good oils. If you have a cook, ration out the oil on a daily or weekly basis.

6. Don't live against the clock

a. Stick to a regular schedule.
b. Eat 2–3 hours before you go to bed.
c. Most social activities revolve around food, so plan your day accordingly.
d. Get good sleep. Avoid large meals before sleeping as they can disrupt sleep, cause discomfort and heartburn. If eating late at night, take a short walk after your meal. Eat 3–4 hours before you go to bed.

7. Shop smart

a. Plan your shopping in advance.
b. Develop the habit of reading labels as you walk down the aisle of a supermarket. Do not buy foods only on the basis of claims such as 'fat-free', 'sugar-free' or 'cholesterol-free'. Buy and stock appropriate snacks like nuts, seeds, fresh fruits, vegetables and roasted foods. Avoid storing unhealthy foods.
c. Read food labels carefully and compare various products on the shelf on the basis of their nutritive value. Pay special attention to the calories, sugar and fat content of foods.
d. Look for hidden fats and sugars on the label and choose foods that are without trans fats and low in sugar and saturated fats.
e. Go organic whenever possible; choose organically or locally grown foods. (See section on reading food labels, p. 90.)
f. A smart shopping list is important; include healthy choices and a variety of nutritious foods.

8. Exercise

a. Engage in regular physical activity for at least 45 minutes, ideally 60 minutes on most days of the week.
b. Hydrate yourself well pre- and post-gym/exercise; drink enough fluids/water. Salted lemon water and coconut water are good options.
c. If you are doing light weights, ensure you have a combination of protein- and carbohydrate-rich snacks like milkshakes, smoothies, fruits, eggs, milk or a cheese/chicken/egg sandwich as soon as you finish.

d. Ensure your diet includes an adequate combination of proteins and carbohydrates for recovery.
e. People tend to feel hungry right after exercising. When managing post-exercise hunger pangs, timing is critical—the sooner you eat after exercising, the better it is. Eating within the first 10 minutes after exercising is better than half an hour, and half an hour is much better than 3 hours.

9. Manage stress

a. Five–ten minutes (during any time of the day) of regular meditation can help you gain control, and clarity of thoughts.
b. Deep-breathing exercises can be done anywhere—in the car, for example—and can help you relax and calm your nerves.
c. Prayer, bio-feedback, neuro-feedback, hypnotherapy and the pursuit of your hobbies are useful stress-management techniques.

10. Have regular health check-ups

a. Follow up on check-ups on a biannual or annual basis. These should include a thorough physical examination, blood pressure measurement, and assessment of blood glucose level, fasting lipid profile, body composition, diet, exercise habits and stress levels.

SOME IMPORTANT HEALTH MARKERS

Body mass index (kg/m^2) <23

Blood pressure (mm/hg) <120/80

Haemoglobin (gm/dl) male ≥13; female ≥12

Total cholesterol (mg/dl) = 150–200

LDL (mg/dl) <100

b. If all is well, such check-ups should be done at least once every 2 years. If any abnormality is found, frequent follow-ups are desirable.

HDL (mg/dl)
male >40; female >50

Triglycerides (mg/dl) <150

Blood glucose
(gm/dl) <100

11. Check medication

a. Continue taking your supplements under the supervision of a qualified practitioner.
b. Losing weight and adopting a healthy lifestyle may require cutting back on medication. Check with your doctor.

12. Don't be tech-shy

Log on to authentic, reliable websites and online weight-management portals like theweightmonitor.com, etc. to help you through your journey, but be careful of not falling into the fad-diet trap. They can help you track your food intake and progress with just a click. Remember, they are only a support and should not become self-treating tools.

13. Your mind counts too

There is a lot of 'mind' in 'food'. Many behavioural issues occur due to deep-set emotional problems and unresolved conflicts. Check your diet, exercise, thoughts and habits like addiction, cravings, alcohol, eating disorders, etc. which conflict with your health goals. Work to correct these, and seek professional help if necessary.

14. Be the change

a. Good eating habits are infectious. You should take the lead and be an example for your family and friends.
b. Involve your family and friends—seek their support when possible. Insensitivity on the part of family members can cause patients to topple over.
c. Do not succumb to social pressures. Learn the art of saying 'no'. Find desirable alternatives.

15. Remember: it's the journey, not the destination

There is no miracle or permanent diet solution for weight management. The benefits will last as long as you follow healthy habits. So make eating healthy a way of life. Here's to a superb journey. Bon voyage!

8

RECIPES

✚ THE DOCTOR SAYS

I am providing here a selection of recipes that connect back to some of the things I have talked about in the book. While I have suggested that you have your regular food for all meals, I have provided here recipes that incorporate raw vegetables; these might be less easy to include. Snacks and desserts often constitute the danger zone for dieters and here are some healthy options for you. To make things even simpler, I have included food groups and serving sizes under each recipe.

Breakfast

SLIMMER'S FIBRE DELIGHT

FOOD GROUP: 1 GRAIN + ½ VEGETABLE

SERVES 6

A hugely filling, low-glycaemic breakfast which gives you the goodness of grains without starch, while incorporating vegetables. A great substitute to poha and upma.

Ingredients

1 tbsp cooking oil, preferably canola oil
1 tsp mustard seeds
3 tbsp curry leaves
1 cup red bell peppers, chopped
1 tbsp (medium) green chillies, deseeded and sliced
1 tsp ginger paste
Salt to taste
1 cup boiled vegetables, finely chopped (carrots, peas, broccoli, red bell peppers, etc.)
1 cup fibre cereal (½ cup oat bran + ½ cup wheat bran)
½ cup water
3 tbsp peanuts, roasted and chopped

Method

1. Heat oil gently over medium flame and add mustard seeds.
2. When the seeds splutter, add the rest of the ingredients except the cereal and peanuts. Cook for about a minute.
3. Add the cereal and roast for a few minutes. Add as much water as needed to achieve an upma-like consistency. Cook for a few more minutes.
4. Add chopped peanuts and serve hot. Serve with fresh green/garlic/coconut/tomato chutney.

Variation: This dish can be enriched with a combination of seeds like sesame, flax, sunflower, etc.

Breakfast

QUINOA VEGETABLE PORRIDGE

FOOD GROUP: 1 GRAIN + 1 VEGETABLE

SERVES 6–8

A low-glycaemic, high-protein breakfast that keeps you going for long. A great substitute to poha or upma.

Ingredients

2 tsp oil, preferably olive oil
½ tsp cumin seeds (jeera)
⅓ cup onions, finely chopped
2 cups mixed vegetables, finely chopped (carrots, cabbage, spinach, peas, beans, baby corn, red bell peppers, etc.; choose any four colours)
½ cup quinoa, cooked
Salt to taste
¼ tsp black pepper
1 tbsp coriander leaves/ parsley, finely chopped

Method

1. Heat oil in a saucepan. Roast cumin seeds for a few seconds and add onion. Cook till translucent.
2. Add chopped vegetables and cook for a few minutes.
3. Add quinoa, salt, pepper and 1 cup water.
4. Cover the saucepan and cook over low heat for about 15 minutes or until quinoa is done. Alternatively, pressure-cook for one whistle.
5. Garnish with fresh coriander or parsley and serve hot.
6. A tangy chutney/relish makes a great accompaniment.

Variation: Quinoa may be substituted with barley. The tempering may be made with mustard and curry leaves, for a south Indian twist.

Breakfast

SAVOURY VEGETABLE 'N' LENTIL BITES

FOOD GROUP: 1 PULSE + ½ VEGETABLE

SERVES 6–8

Makes for an excellent low-fat, high-nutrient and filling breakfast or evening snack.

Ingredients

Savoury bites

1 cup gram flour/lentil flour
2 tbsp oat bran/wheat bran
2 tbsp fenugreek leaves, chopped/2 tbsp dried fenugreek powder (kasuri methi)
1 tbsp green chillies, chopped (optional)
1 tsp cumin seeds
½ tsp turmeric powder (haldi)
½ tsp sugar
1 tsp lemon juice
Salt to taste
2 tbsp cooking oil
4 cups cabbage, very finely shredded

Tempering

2 tbsp oil
½ tsp mustard seeds

Method

1. Combine gram flour, oat or wheat bran, fenugreek, green chillies (if using), cumin seeds, turmeric powder, sugar, lemon juice, oil and salt in a bowl.
2. Add shredded cabbage and blend well. The mixture should be like a very soft dough.
3. Divide the mixture with greased fingers into 14 pcs and drop them into the steamer. Cover and steam for about 18–20 minutes. Savoury bites are done when a knife put through them comes out clean.
4. When cool, cut each piece into half.
5. For tempering, heat oil in a frying pan over medium flame. Add mustard seeds. When they splutter, add sesame seeds and red chillies and stir-fry for a few seconds.

1 tbsp sesame seeds
4 red chillies

Garnish
2 tbsp coriander leaves, chopped

6. Add savoury bites and stir-fry for a few minutes until they are light brown.
7. Garnish with chopped coriander leaves.

Notes:

1. Make the mixture just before you are ready to steam. Otherwise the mixture will leave water and will become very soft. If you're making more than one batch, add salt one batch at a time.
2. Savoury bites may be refrigerated for 3–4 days and may also be frozen.

Variation: Cabbage may be substituted with zucchini or bottle gourd. As these vegetables have more water content, after shredding lightly squeeze them between your palms to get the excess water out before making the mixture. Fenugreek may be substituted with curry leaves.

Breakfast

BROWN-RICE PANCAKES

FOOD GROUP: 1 GRAIN + ½ VEGETABLE

SERVES 4

SIZE OF SERVING: 2 PANCAKES

Great substitute to conventional pancakes. Good for breakfast or main course. Treat 1 medium-sized pancake as 1 serving of grains/cereals.

Ingredients

1 cup brown-rice flour
¼ cup skimmed milk
1½ cups spinach, finely chopped
¼ cup onions, very finely chopped
1 tsp garlic, crushed
¼ tsp green chillies, chopped (optional)
Salt to taste
Red chilli powder to taste
Cooking oil

Method

1. Mix brown-rice flour in the milk. The mixture should have a pouring consistency. Add more milk/water if the mixture feels too thick.
2. Add spinach, onions, garlic and green chillies. Season with salt and red chilli powder.
3. Heat a non-stick pan and spread the batter with a round spoon.
4. Spoon oil around the pancake. Let the pancake brown on one side.
5. Remove from pan. Serve hot with a chutney and stuffing of choice if desired.

Stuffing suggestions

1. Mushrooms and onions, finely chopped and sautéed.
2. Moong sprouts, lightly sautéed, with crushed peanuts.
3. Cottage cheese/tofu, mashed seasoned and sautéed.

Variation: Brown-rice flour may be substituted with oat flour, or you could just grind brown rice in a dry grinder. A combination of canola, rice-bran, cold-pressed sesame, mustard and extra virgin olive oils may be used. They are all healthy oils.

Breakfast

MOONG DAL POHA

FOOD GROUP: 1 PULSE

SERVES 2

Also called 'sundal' in south India. A low–glycaemic index, low-carbohydrate breakfast which keeps you full for long. Count it under your pulse allowance.

Ingredients

- ½ cup peas, shelled
- A pinch of sugar
- Salt to taste
- 1 cup moong dal, split and soaked for 1 hour
- ½ tsp cooking oil
- ½ tsp black-mustard seeds
- ½ tsp ginger, finely chopped
- ½ tbsp green chillies, finely chopped (optional)
- 1 tbsp curry leaves, finely chopped
- ¼ cup coriander leaves
- ½ cup onions, finely chopped
- ½ cup tomatoes, finely chopped
- ¼ tsp red chilli powder (optional)
- ¼ tsp turmeric powder (optional)

Method

1. Boil peas in a small bowl with 1½ cups of water, a pinch of sugar and salt to taste.
2. Wash dal; add salt and 2 cups of water. Boil till done.
3. Heat oil in a pan, add mustard seeds and allow them to splutter. Add ginger and green chillies(if using) and cook for about a minute.
4. Add curry leaves and sauté for 2–3 minutes.
5. Add dal and peas, and blend well. Mix in red chilli powder and turmeric powder (if using).
6. Add coriander leaves, onions and tomatoes. Cook for about a minute or until done.
7. Garnish with curry leaves and serve hot.

Beverages

FRUIT SMOOTHIE

FOOD GROUP: 1½ FRUITS + 1 DAIRY

SERVES 1

Ideal as a post–workout energizer.

Ingredients

Smoothie

1½ cups yogurt
¾ cup seasonal fruits, mashed (bananas, mangoes, strawberries, papaya, kiwis, chiku, etc.)
1 tsp sugar (optional)
⅓ cup ice, crushed

Garnish

1 tbsp seasonal fruits, chopped

Method

1. Put yogurt, fruits and sugar in a blender with ice. Blend until smooth.
2. Pour into a tall glass and garnish with chopped fruits.
3. Serve chilled.

Beverages

APPLE AND STRAWBERRY SMOOTHIE

FOOD GROUP: 1 FRUIT + ½ DAIRY

SERVES 1

Ideal as a breakfast beverage.

Ingredients

6–8 strawberries
½ cup apple juice
½ cup low-fat yogurt
1 tsp fresh mint leaves

Method

1. Cook the strawberries in a little water until soft and then drain.
2. Blend well with apple juice and then add yogurt.
3. Garnish with fresh mint leaves.

Variation: You can substitute yogurt with milk or soy milk.

FIG SHAKE

FOOD GROUP: 1 FRUIT + 1 DAIRY

SERVES 1

Ideal as an evening snack.

Ingredients

3 dried figs
1½ cups apple juice
¼ tsp cloves, ground (optional)
½ tsp almond extract

Method

1. Blend all ingredients in a blender.
2. Serve chilled.

Beverages

VEGETABLE JUICE

FOOD GROUP: 2–3 VEGETABLES

SERVES 5

A power-packed beverage which can make a huge difference to your weight, health and well-being. It also helps train your taste buds.

Ingredients

1 cup cucumbers, peeled and cubed
1 cup tomatoes, chopped
1 cup carrots, peeled and cubed
2 cups white gourd, peeled and cubed
½ cup beetroot, peeled and cubed
2 tbsp celery, chopped
1" stick fresh turmeric
4 amlas, deseeded/1 tbsp lemon juice (optional)
½ tsp black salt
½ tsp cumin powder
1 bunch coriander leaves/ mint leaves, torn

Method

1. Run the vegetables through a juicer.
2. Season with lemon juice (if using), black salt and cumin powder.
3. Garnish with coriander or mint leaves and serve cold.

Snacks

SOY CUTLETS

FOOD GROUP: 1 PULSE

SERVES 4–6

A great way to incorporate soy, which has a low glycaemic index. Ideal for breakfast, kids' tiffin or evening snack.

Ingredients

½ cup soy granules
2 tsp soy oil
1 tsp coriander seeds
1 tsp ginger paste
1 tsp garlic paste
1 tbsp green chillies, chopped
½ tsp red chilli powder
I tbsp coriander powder
1 tsp turmeric power
1½ cups potatoes, boiled, peeled and mashed
Salt to taste
¾ cup breadcrumbs
Oil for deep frying, preferably soy oil
2 tbsp coriander leaves

Method

1. Soak soy granules in water for 15 minutes. Squeeze to remove excess water.
2. Heat oil in a pan and add coriander seeds. When they splutter, add ginger paste, garlic paste and chopped green chillies; stir for a moment.
3. Add red chilli powder, coriander powder and turmeric powder while stirring continuously. Then add soy granules and cook till granules are cooked and dry.
4. Add potatoes, adjust salt and continue cooking till the mixture completely dries up. Remove the pan from heat and allow it to cool. Add coriander leaves.
5. Now add breadcrumbs and mix well. Divide into small, equal portions and shape each portion into a cutlet. Deep-fry in moderately hot oil until crisp. Serve hot.

Snacks

FALAFEL

FOOD GROUP: 1 PULSE

SERVES 6

Traditional Middle Eastern kebabs made with chickpeas. Traditionally fried, but should not be allowed to absorb in too much oil. May be grilled.

Ingredients

1 cup chickpeas, soaked overnight
1 cup spring onions, chopped
1 tbsp garlic, chopped
4 (large) sprigs parsley
Salt to taste
Black pepper to taste
½ tsp cumin powder
1 tsp coriander powder
Cooking oil for deep-frying

Method

1. Drain the chickpeas and combine with spring onions, garlic, parsley and 3 tbsp of water in an electric blender or food processor. Blend to a purée, scraping down the sides when necessary. Add cumin powder, coriander powder, and salt and pepper to taste. Then transfer into a bowl and leave for 1–2 hours to dry out slightly.
2. Divide the mixture into walnut-sized balls and flatten these slightly. Heat the oil in a deep-fryer, add the falafel and fry for about 4 minutes or until golden. Drain on kitchen paper.
3. Serve hot with salad, yogurt dip or hummus.

Variation: Falafel may also be pan-fried or roasted.

Snacks

COTTAGE CHEESE OR TOFU TIKKI

FOOD GROUP: 1 DAIRY + 1 VEGETABLE

SERVES 4

A high-protein, calcium-rich and filling snack, especially for vegetarians. Great for breakfast, kids' tiffin or meals.

Ingredients

1 cup cottage cheese/tofu, mashed
½ cup peas, shelled and boiled
½ cup carrots, boiled
1 tsp green chillies, chopped
A few sprigs coriander leaves
½ tsp garlic paste
½ tsp black pepper
Cooking oil for frying

Method

1. Combine all the ingredients and mix well.
2. Divide the mixture into flat, round balls and shallow-fry or bake the tikkis, using only a little oil.
3. Serve hot with coriander chutney.

Snacks

INSTANT DHOKLA

FOOD GROUP: 1 PULSE

SERVES 4

Popular traditional Indian breakfast or evening snack. Very low in fat and has a low glycaemic index. May be made with different pulse flours, oats or quinoa flour.

Ingredients

Dhokla

1 cup gram flour
1 cup yogurt
1 tsp sugar
1 tsp salt
2 tsp Eno's Fruit Salt
½ tsp baking soda
2 tsp oil, preferably canola oil

Tempering

2 tsp oil, preferably canola oil
½ tsp mustard seeds
½ tsp sesame seeds
½ tbsp green chillies, chopped
1 sprig curry leaves
1 tbsp lemon juice

Method

Dhokla

1. Combine all ingredients except oil and the tempering ingredients in a bowl.
2. Set aside for 30 minutes to ferment.
3. Add oil to the fermented batter and beat well.
4. Spread batter in a lightly greased tin or thali with raised edges.
5. Steam for 10 minutes. Remove from heat, allow to cool, cut into squares and arrange on a serving dish.

Tempering

1. Heat oil for tempering in a small pan. Add mustard seeds and when they splutter, add remaining tempering ingredients. Stir for a minute and pour contents of pan over dhokla.
2. Serve hot or cold.

Soups

BROCCOLI SOUP

FOOD GROUP: 1 VEGETABLE + ½ CEREAL

SERVES 4

A great way to fill up, this dish can be made into a meal soup.

Ingredients

2½ cups broccoli
2 tsp olive oil
1 cup onions, sliced
2 tsp garlic, finely chopped
2½ cups potatoes, peeled and sliced
6 cups vegetable stock/water
1 cup low-fat milk
⅛ tsp salt
⅛ tsp black pepper

Method

1. Cut the broccoli florets from the stems. Using a vegetable peeler, peel the broccoli stems, then slice them.
2. In a large saucepan, heat oil over moderate heat. Sauté onions and garlic until soft. Add ½ cup of water and cook for about 5 minutes. Add broccoli stems to the saucepan with potatoes, stock and milk. Partially cover the saucepan and simmer for about 8–10 minutes or until broccoli and potatoes are tender.
3. Stir in the broccoli florets and simmer for 5 more minutes or until the florets are very tender.
4. Remove from heat. With a skimmer or slotted spoon, transfer the vegetables to a blender or food processor. Purée until very smooth.
5. Return purée to the liquid in the saucepan. Return the pan to heat until the soup is warmed through. Season with salt and pepper.

Soups

CARROT SOUP

FOOD GROUP: 1 VEGETABLE

SERVES 4

Makes for a complete meal when combined with a protein- or grain-/cereal-based preparation.

Ingredients

- 1 tsp unsalted butter or olive oil
- 1 cup onions, sliced
- 2½ cups carrots, chopped
- 2 tbsp tomato paste
- ¼ cup rice
- 6–8 cups vegetable stock
- Salt to taste
- Black pepper to taste, freshly ground
- ¾ cup milk

Method

1. Heat butter or olive oil in a heavy soup pot. Add sliced onions and sauté. Add carrots and sauté till almost tender.
2. Add tomato paste, rice and 4 cups of vegetable stock, and simmer for about 25 minutes or until everything is very tender.
3. Purée in a blender or food processor. Return the soup to the pot and add additional stock. Season with salt and pepper. Simmer for 5 more minutes. Pour in the milk and heat through. Serve hot.

Soups

COLD CUCUMBER AND MINT SOUP

FOOD GROUP: 2 VEGETABLES

SERVES 3–4

An excellent way to add the raw-food quotient to your diet.

Ingredients

1½ cups cucumber, peeled and diced
1½ cups spring onions, trimmed and chopped
3 tbsp yogurt
1 tbsp lemon juice
2 tpsp mint leaves, finely chopped
Salt to taste
Black pepper to taste, freshly ground

Method

1. In a blender, combine cucumber, spring onions and 2¼ cups of water. Blend together until smooth.
2. Add yogurt and lemon juice.
3. Stir mint leaves into yogurt mixture.
4. Season to taste.
5. Refrigerate and serve cold.
6. Garnish with mint.

Soups

SUMMER SOUP I

FOOD GROUP: 2 VEGETABLES

SERVES 3–4

A truly refreshing version of a raw vegetable juice, this soup helps to keep you full and your digestion well oiled.

Ingredients

Soup

1½ cups cucumber, coarsely chopped
5 cups tomatoes, peeled, deseeded and halved
½ cup onions, finely chopped
½ cup green bell peppers, deseeded and chopped
1 tsp garlic paste
1¼ cups chicken stock
Salt to taste
Black pepper to taste
1 tsp sugar
3 tbsp vinegar

Garnish

1 cup cucumber, diced
1 tbsp parsley, finely chopped

Method

1. Purée vegetables in a blender or by pushing through a sieve.
2. Stir stock, salt, black pepper, sugar and vinegar into the purée.
3. Chill for a few hours.
4. Garnish with diced cucumber and parsley.
5. Serve cold.

Soups

SUMMER SOUP II

FOOD GROUP: 1 DAIRY + 2 VEGETABLES

SERVES 3–4

A great starter.

Ingredients

Soup
1½ cups tomato purée
1 cup yogurt
1 cup milk, cold
½ tbsp lemon juice
1 tsp sugar, powdered
1 tsp celery, finely chopped
1 tsp spring onions, finely chopped
Salt to taste
Black pepper to taste

Garnish
2 tbsp parsley, chopped

Method

1. Mix all the ingredients together.
2. Put into individual soup bowls.
3. Garnish with parsley.
4. Serve cold.

Salads

BROCCOLI AND SESAME SALAD

FOOD GROUP: 1 VEGETABLE

SERVES 4

Loaded with antioxidants, sesame adds taste and nutrition. Low in carbohydrates, this dish makes for a great filling salad.

Ingredients

Salad

1 cup broccoli, cut into small florets and steamed
½ cup bell peppers, sliced
1 cup iceberg lettuce/Chinese cabbage, torn and coarsely chopped

Dressing

2 tsp light soy sauce
2 tbsp white-wine vinegar/lemon juice
2 tsp sesame oil/peanut oil
1 tbsp honey
1 tbsp sesame seeds, lightly roasted
Salt to taste
White pepper to taste

Method

1. Combine vegetables in a bowl. Set aside.
2. Combine ingredients for dressing. Mix well or shake in a bottle till well blended.
3. Pour dressing over salad.
4. Toss lightly and serve.

Salads

RAW PAPAYA SALAD

FOOD GROUP: 1 VEGETABLE

SERVES 4

A truly light yet satisfying salad, great for summers.

Ingredients

2 cups raw papaya, grated
½ cup peanuts, chopped
½ cup tomatoes, sliced
½ cup spring onions, chopped
½ cup bean sprouts (optional)
¼ cup coriander leaves

Dressing
1 tsp salt
1 tbsp honey or sugar
1 tsp chilli flakes
3 tbsp light soy sauce
¼ cup lemon juice
1½ tsp garlic paste

Method

1. Combine dressing ingredients in a cup.
2. Combine grated papaya, tomatoes, spring onion, bean sprouts (if using), coriander leaves and most of the peanuts (saving some for the garnish).
3. Pour the dressing on to the vegetables and toss well.
4. Garnish with fresh coriander leaves and chopped peanuts.

Variation: Raw mangoes, cucumber or raw apples can be used in place of raw papaya.

Salads

FRUIT 'N' NUT COLESLAW SALAD

FOOD GROUP: 1 FRUIT + ½ NUTS

SERVES 4

The nuts, raisins and apricots make this an unusual coleslaw. It is filling and has a low glycaemic index.

Ingredients

Salad
2½ cups cabbage, shredded
¾ cup carrots, grated
¾ cup dried apricots, seeded and coarsely chopped
¾ cup walnuts, coarsely chopped
¾ cup seedless raisins
2 tbsp fresh parsley, chopped

Dressing
7 tbsp mayonnaise
5 tbsp yogurt, whisked smooth
1¼ tsp salt
½ tsp black pepper

Garnish
1 cup apples, sliced

Method

1. Combine all salad ingredients in a salad bowl. Toss to mix.
2. In a separate bowl, mix mayonnaise and yogurt. Season to taste with salt and black pepper.
3. Add dressing to salad and toss till salad is well coated.
4. Cover the bowl and set aside in the refrigerator for at least 30 minutes before serving, to allow the flavours to blend.
5. Garnish with apple slices and serve.

Salads

BALI VEGETABLE SALAD WITH PEANUT DRESSING

FOOD GROUP: 2 DAIRY + 1 VEGETABLE + ½ NUTS

SERVES 4

A great blend of vegetables. Use any combination of seasonal vegetables; sprouts, tofu and peanuts add good plant protein.

Ingredients

Salad

¾ cup tofu (extra firm), cut into 1" cubes
Cooking oil for greasing
2 tbsp light soy sauce
6 cups mixed baby salad greens
1 cup green beans, lightly blanched
¾ cup carrots, peeled and julienned
2 (medium) tomatoes, cut into 4 wedges
1 cup moong bean sprouts
¾ cup cucumber, peeled, seeded and sliced in moons

Dressing

½ cup tofu (firm), mashed
3 tbsp peanut butter
2 tbsp light soy sauce

Method

1. Pat dry the defrosted tofu with paper towels.
2. Grease a non-stick grill pan or a cast-iron skillet with cooking oil.
3. Grill tofu for 3–4 minutes on each side.
4. Drizzle soy sauce over tofu during the last 30 seconds of cooking time. Reserve.
5. Combine the dressing ingredients in a blender and blend until smooth and creamy.
6. Mix greens with half of the dressing.
7. Arrange tofu on top and garnish with green beans, tomatoes, carrots, sprouts and cucumber. Serve with additional dressing and garnish with coriander leaves.

5 tbsp rice vinegar
2 tbsp maple syrup/honey
1 tbsp unrefined cane sugar
1 tbsp fresh ginger, peeled and chopped
¼ tsp red chilli flakes (optional)
4 tbsp light, unsweetened coconut milk
½ cup spring onions, finely chopped

Garnish
¼ cup fresh coriander leaves

Salads

SALAD WITH PESTO SAUCE

FOOD GROUP: 2 VEGETABLES + 1 NUTS

SERVES 4

The simplest salad pesto. This dish makes for a substantial salad and a complete meal.

Ingredients

Salad

5 cups lettuce, torn
1½ cups carrots, steamed and sliced
1½ cups green beans, stringed and cut in to 2" pcs
1½ cups mushrooms, steamed and chopped
1½ cups cauliflower florets, steamed
¼ cup tomatoes, sliced
1½ cups broccoli florets, steamed (optional)
1¼ cups black and green olives, sliced

Dressing (Basil pesto sauce)

12 cloves garlic
½ cup cashews
¾ cup basil leaves, finely chopped
3 tbsp olive oil
Salt to taste
Black pepper to taste, freshly ground

Method

1. Arrange lettuce in a flat, shallow bowl. Place vegetables (except olives) on it such that vegetables of contrasting colours are next to each other.
2. For the pesto sauce, blend the ingredients into a thick, green cream, using a food processor or blender.
3. Sprinkle chopped olives and pour pesto sauce on the vegetables.
4. Serve immediately.

Note: The combination of vegetables can be varied according to availability as long as you include different colours.

Dressings

SIMPLE OIL AND VINEGAR DRESSING

MAKES ¾ CUP

An all-time favourite, this basic dressing can be used with just about any salad.

Ingredients

¼ cup rice vinegar
½ tsp sea salt
¼ tsp black pepper, freshly ground
1 tsp garlic, minced or chopped
½ tsp dry basil
1 tsp brown-rice syrup, honey or apple concentrate
½ cup oil, preferably olive oil

Method

1. Whisk all the ingredients except the oil together in a small jar.
2. Add the oil and mix well.
3. Store in refrigerator.

Dressings

PARSLEY AND PUMPKIN-SEED DRESSING

MAKES 1½ –2 CUPS

An unusual seed-based dressing.

Ingredients

3 cups or 1 bunch fresh parsley, chopped
¼ cup pumpkin seeds
½ tsp sea salt
2½ tbsp lemon juice
1 clove garlic
1 tbsp olive oil

Method

1. Put all ingredients in a blender with half a cup of water and blend until smooth.
2. Store in refrigerator.

Dressings

CORIANDER GREEN GODDESS DRESSING

MAKES 1½–2 CUPS

A highly nutritious dressing which can line any salad.

Ingredients

½ cup tofu (firm), mashed
½ cup spring onions, chopped
2 tbsp fresh lemon juice
½ cup fresh parsley, chopped
¼ cup fresh cilantro leaves, chopped
1 tbsp honey
¼ cup apple cider vinegar
1 tsp Worcestershire sauce, vegetarian
1 tsp prepared mustard
1 tsp fresh jalapeno chilli, minced (optional)

Method

1. Combine ingredients in a blender.
2. Blend until smooth and creamy.
3. Store in refrigerator.

Main course

HERBED CHICKEN WITH MANGO

FOOD GROUP: ½ LEAN MEAT + ½ VEGETABLE + ½ FRUIT

SERVES 4

An interesting variation to the conventional roast chicken.

Ingredients

4 chicken breasts, boneless and skinless
2 tsp herbs
2 tbsp olive oil (divided)
2 cups onions, thinly sliced
2 cups mangoes, diced
4 tbsp low-fat feta cheese, crumbled

Method

1. Preheat oven to 190–200°C.
2. Rub each chicken breast with herbs.
3. In a large, oven-proof skillet, heat ½ tbsp olive oil and add chicken. Cook chicken for 2–3 minutes a side or till light golden.
4. Add remaining oil and sliced onions. Continue to cook until onions are translucent.
5. Lightly cover the skillet with foil. Place skillet in the oven and bake chicken and onions for about 15 minutes. Chicken should reach 75°C when tested with a thermometer.
6. Remove from oven. Let rest (still covered) for about 5 minutes before serving.
7. Plate chicken as follows: make a bed of cooked onion and place chicken breasts on top. Arrange diced mangoes on and around chicken. Sprinkle each with a tablespoon or two of feta cheese. Serve hot.

Variation: Mangoes may be substituted with boiled, chopped and cubed pumpkin.

Main course

GRILLED PEPPER CHICKEN IN CREAM CHEESE

FOOD GROUP: 1 LEAN MEAT + ½ DAIRY

SERVES 4–6

A simple, healthy and quick way to do chicken.

Ingredients

4 chicken breasts, halved and flattened

Marinade

1 cup hung curd
⅓ cup mayonnaise
1½ tsp garlic paste
Salt to taste
1 tsp chilli flakes
1 tsp white pepper
1 tsp olive oil

Method

1. Combine marinade ingredients.
2. Marinate chicken breasts for about 30 minutes and cook on a grill for 7–8 minutes or until done.
3. The chicken may also be pan-fried or put into a foil and baked for 10–12 minutes.
4. Serve hot.

Main course

BAKED FLAX 'N' HERB CHICKEN ROLLS

FOOD GROUP: 2 LEAN MEATS

SERVES 6–8

Completely oil-free and loaded with vegetables.

Ingredients

2 tsp garlic paste
Salt to taste
Black pepper to taste
4 chicken breasts, sliced cross-wise to make 8 flat pcs
¾ cup apple juice
¾ cup white wine

Filling

¾ cup quinoa/barley/brown rice, cooked
¼ cup onions, sliced and golden fried
¼ cup parsley, chopped
¼ cup flaxseeds, ground
1 tsp ginger paste
Salt to taste
Red chilli powder to taste

Method

1. Rub garlic paste, salt and pepper on to chicken breasts and lay them flat.
2. Combine the ingredients for the filling. Season to taste.
3. Place 2 tbsp of filling on each breast and roll it up. Secure well; use toothpick if needed. Place in a baking dish.
4. Pour apple juice and white wine over the chicken and bake for 20–30 minutes at 180°C. The rolls can also be wrapped individually in foil and baked the same way.

Main course

PAN-FRIED COTTAGE CHEESE WITH CHILLI–GARLIC SAUCE

FOOD GROUP: 1 DAIRY + 1 VEGETABLE

SERVES 4

Cottage cheese is immensely filling and adds much-needed calcium to your daily diet.

Ingredients

3 tsp olive oil
2 tbsp garlic, chopped
1 cup spring onions, chopped
1 tbsp chilli sauce
1 tbsp soy sauce
1 cup cottage cheese, cubed
Salt to taste
White pepper to taste
A pinch of sugar (optional)

Method

1. Heat oil over medium flame. Add garlic and spring onions. Cook for about a minute till onions are lightly cooked.
2. Add the rest of the ingredients. Stir-fry for a few minutes till heated through.
3. Serve hot.

Main course

PAN-FRIED TOFU WITH GREENS

FOOD GROUP: 1 PULSE + 3 VEGETABLES

SERVES 4

A simple, conventional tofu dish with sesame, peanuts and tangy soy sauce. It is a filling main course and, combined with a cereal, makes for a complete meal.

Ingredients

1 cup tofu, sliced into 2" pcs
Oil for pan-frying, preferably canola oil
1 cup spring onions, chopped
1 cup pak choy
1 cup Chinese greens
2 cups spinach
1 cup Chinese cabbage

Marinade

1 tsp salt
2 tsp peanut oil/canola oil
2 tsp sesame oil, toasted
1" stick ginger, crushed
4 cloves garlic, crushed
1 tsp white pepper
3 tbsp vinegar/red wine
2 tbsp brown sugar/4 tsp honey
4 tbsp dark soy sauce
2 tbsp tomato ketchup

Method

1. Combine all marinade ingredients. Add sliced tofu and set aside for a few minutes.
2. Heat oil in a shallow, non-stick pan.
3. Remove tofu from marinade.
4. Pan-fry gently till golden. Keep aside.
5. Add more oil to the pan. Add sesame seeds and cook for a minute or two till light golden.
6. Add the greens. Stir-fry rapidly on high heat till just cooked. (Overcooking will cause water to drain out of leaves and make them limp.)
7. Season with salt, pepper and brown sugar.
8. To the remaining marinade, add the tomato ketchup and bring it to a boil till it thickens to a sauce.
9. Arrange greens on a flat serving dish. Arrange cooked tofu. Pour sauce over it. Serve hot.

Seasoning for greens
4 tsp sesame seeds
1 tsp salt
1 tsp white pepper
2 tsp brown sugar

Variation: Seasonal vegetables of your choice and cottage cheese may be used as a variation.

Main course

ROASTED VEGETABLES

FOOD GROUP: 2 VEGETABLES

SERVES 4

The easiest non-cereal/grain evening meal. It is quite light and takes care of your cooked-vegetable quota.

Ingredients

½ cup red bell peppers, cubed
½ cup green bell peppers, cubed
½ cup yellow bell peppers, cubed
½ cup broccoli florets
½ cup zucchini, sliced
½ cup mushrooms, halved
1 (medium) onion, quartered
1 tbsp cooking oil, preferably olive oil
2 cloves garlic, crushed
½ tsp salt
¼ tsp black pepper

Dressing

1 tbsp olive oil/canola oil
2 cloves garlic, crushed
1 tsp dried herbs
½ tsp salt
¼ tsp black pepper
1 tbsp vinegar/balsamic/red wine

Method

1. Preheat grill.
2. In a large bowl, combine vegetables with oil, garlic, salt and pepper.
3. Transfer to a non-stick baking dish and roast, stirring occasionally, for about 7–10 minutes.
4. Remove from grill and transfer to a bowl.
5. Combine dressing ingredients.
6. Toss the vegetables, while still hot, in the dressing.

Variation: Garlic mayonnaise (aioli) may also be used instead of the dressing.

Main course

KHAO-SUEY

FOOD GROUP: 2 LEAN MEATS + 1 NUTS

SERVES 4

This all-time Burmese meal soup is hugely filling, even without rice or noodles.

Ingredients

500 gm chicken, whole
½ cup onions, finely chopped
½" stick ginger
12 cloves garlic
1 tbsp oil, preferably canola oil
2 tbsp chickpea flour
¾ tsp turmeric powder
2½ cups coconut milk
½ tsp salt
½ tsp black pepper
½ tsp garam masala

Garnish

3 tbsp garlic, golden fried
3 tbsp onions, sliced, golden fried
3 tbsp spring onions, finely chopped
3 tbsp coriander leaves, finely chopped
3 tbsp pink onions, finely chopped

Method

1. Boil chicken in 1 tsp salt and 7 cups of water for at least 1–2 hours (the longer the better). Alternatively, pressure-cook for one whistle, lower the heat and cook for another 30 minutes. Cool, debone and shred chicken finely. Reserve stock.
2. In a food processor, grind onions, ginger and garlic to a paste. Pan-fry paste in oil till reddish brown.
3. Lower the heat and add chickpea flour and turmeric powder. Cook on low heat for 2–3 minutes. Add coconut milk and boil till the mixture thickens.
4. Blend the mixture well and add to the chicken stock with chicken shreds. Simmer the broth till it thickens. Adjust consistency with water if too thick.
5. Remove from heat. Season with salt, black pepper and garam masala.

3 tbsp green chillies, deseeded and finely chopped
3 tbsp lemon juice
1 egg, boiled and finely chopped
1 tsp red chilli sauce (optional)
1 tbsp sesame seeds, toasted
1 tbsp peanuts, roasted

6. Serve in soup bowls, garnished with garlic cloves, sliced onions, spring onions, coriander leaves, chopped onions, green chillies, fried garlic cloves, lemon juice, boiled egg, red chilli sauce (if using), toasted sesame seeds and roasted peanuts.

Main course

CHICKEN ROULADE

FOOD GROUP: 1 LEAN MEAT + ½ VEGETABLE

SERVES 6

A visual treat and a welcome change from the usual chicken preparations. Combined with salad/soup/vegetables, it makes for an easy supper maincourse.

Ingredients

2½ cups chicken, minced
½ cups onions, chopped
½ tbsp green chillies, deseeded and finely chopped
1 tsp garlic paste
1 tsp salt (divided)
1 tsp black pepper (divided)
1 tbsp coriander leaves, finely chopped
1 tbsp tomato paste or ketchup
½ cup low-fat cottage cheese
½ cup mushrooms, sautéed
1¼ cups spinach, thawed, drained and chopped
1 cup onions, thinly sliced
1 cup carrots, coarsely chopped
2½ cups tomatoes, crushed
Oil for greasing

Method

1. In a bowl, mix chicken, chopped onions, green chillies, garlic paste, ½ tsp salt, ½ tsp black pepper, coriander leaves, and tomato paste or ketchup.
2. In another bowl, mix cottage cheese, mushrooms, spinach, ½ tsp salt and ½ tsp black pepper.
3. Turn the chicken mixture on to a sheet of butter paper/aluminium foil and form a 9"x10" rectangle with your hands.
4. Spoon the spinach mixture lengthwise down the centre of the chicken, leaving about 1" uncovered at each short end.
5. With the help of the butter paper/foil, lift the long edges of the chicken. Fold the chicken sheet over stuffing to enclose it.
6. Using your fingers, pinch the edges of the chicken roll together.

7. Grease a non-stick pan and put over heat. Place chicken roll seam-side down on the pan and brown surface on all sides, till sealed. Add onions, carrots and tomatoes to the pan.
8. Cover and cook for about 30–45 minutes, until chicken and vegetables are cooked.
9. Transfer chicken to a serving platter. Purée vegetables in a blender and serve as a sauce with the chicken roll.

Main course

PACIFIC TOFU

FOOD GROUP: 1 PULSE + 2 VEGETABLES

SERVES 6

This typical tofu-and-vegetable combination along with bean sprouts is filling and nutritious.

Ingredients

6 tbsp light soy sauce
2 tsp balsamic vinegar
2 tsp honey
1 tbsp rice wine
2 tbsp fresh ginger, peeled and grated
1 tbsp garlic, minced
½ tsp sesame oil, toasted
1 cup tofu (extra firm), cut into 1" cubes
½ cup spring onions, sliced diagonally into 1" pcs
1 tsp sesame oil, toasted
6 cups vegetables, chopped (broccoli, asparagus, green cabbage, red bell peppers, snow peas, bean sprouts, etc.)
Oil for greasing

Method

1. Preheat oven to 200°C.
2. In a small bowl, blend soy sauce, vinegar, honey, rice wine, ginger, garlic and sesame oil until smooth.
3. Coat a baking tray with cooking oil. Pat tofu with paper towels to dry out moisture. Place tofu cubes on the sheet in a single layer. Pour half of the soy sauce mixture over tofu. Bake for 30 minutes.
4. Sauté spring onions and sesame oil in a wok/skillet for a minute; add vegetables and remaining soy sauce mixture.
5. Stir-fry for about 5 minutes. Add cooked tofu and toss lightly.
6. Serve with steamed rice or cooked pasta.

Main course

BEET RAITA

FOOD GROUP: 1 VEGETABLE + ½ DAIRY

SERVES 6

Beetroot is loaded with antioxidants and this delicious raita adds valuable raw vegetables and dairy to your diet.

Ingredients

3 cups beetroot, grated
1 tsp cooking oil
½ tsp mustard seeds
1 tbsp curry leaves, crumbled
1 tsp sea salt
1 tbsp honey,
2 cups yogurt

Method

1. Put an inch of water in a large saucepan and set it in a stainless-steel steamer. Put grated beetroot in the steamer and bring water to boil. Cover and steam beetroot for 2–3 minutes over medium heat.
2. Heat oil in a small skillet. Add mustard seeds and crumbled curry leaves. When the mustard seeds splutter, take the skillet off the heat.
3. Put steamed beetroot, oil, spices and rest of the ingredients in a medium-sized mixing bowl and mix well.
4. Serve cold.

Variation: Beetroot may be substituted with any seasonal vegetable like spinach or other greens.

Desserts

BAKED APPLES

FOOD GROUP: 2 FRUITS

SERVES 4

A simple dessert for that sweet tooth.

Ingredients

4 (medium) apples
½ cup raisins
1 tbsp cinnamon
¼ tsp nutmeg/cardamom
¼ tsp lemon peel/
1 tsp lemon juice
¼ cup sunflower seeds
2 cups apple juice
1 tsp unsalted butter (optional)

Method

1. Preheat the oven to 180°C.
2. Wash and core apples. Place in 8"x8" baking dish.
3. Mix raisins, spices and seeds. Stuff this mixture firmly into the cored apples.
4. Pour apple juice into the pan and dot the centre of each apple with butter (if using).
5. Cover and bake for 45 minutes or until tender.

Desserts

CRISPY GRANOLA

FOOD GROUP: 1 CEREAL + ½ SEED + ½ FRUIT

SERVING SIZE: ¼ CUP OR 3 TBSP

Rich in low-glycaemic whole grains, this household recipe for old-fashioned granola is good for breakfast, and makes a good substitute to bakery, biscuits and rusks.

Ingredients

- 4 cups rolled oats
- 1 cup oat bran
- ½ cup sunflower seeds, ground
- ½ cup sunflower seeds
- ½ cup pumpkin seeds (optional)
- 1–1½ cups raisins
- ½ cup dried apple/dried apricot, chopped (optional)
- 3 tbsp cooking oil
- ¼ cup apple juice
- 2 tbsp cinnamon
- ½ –1 tsp dried ginger
- ¼ tsp cloves, ground

Method

1. Preheat oven to 150°C.
2. Mix the dry ingredients together.
3. Combine oil and apple juice in a separate large bowl and whisk together.
4. Mix in the spices, then add the dry ingredients.
5. Mix well until the oats are coated.
6. Spoon the mixture into one or two large, shallow, ungreased baking dishes.
7. Bake for about 30 minutes or until golden brown. Cool until crisp.

Desserts

APPLE CRUMBLE

FOOD GROUP: ¼ GRAINS/CEREALS + 2 FRUITS

SERVES 4

The whole-grain muesli replaces the white-flour crumble in the conventional recipe, making it healthier. Sugar is substituted with a sweetener which makes for a low-calorie dessert. Feel free to use unrefined sugar in small amounts.

Ingredients

3 cups apples, peeled and thinly sliced
1 tbsp brown sugar
3 sachets sucralose (sugar substitute)
1 tsp cinnamon powder
1½ tsp lemon juice

Crumble

½ cup muesli/granola/whole-grain breakfast cereal
1 tbsp butter

Method

1. Preheat oven to 180°C.
2. Combine apples with brown sugar, sucralose, cinnamon powder and lemon juice. Turn mixture on to a butter pie dish.
3. Combine ingredients for crumble topping. Grind the muesli, if you like a finer texture.
4. Rub muesli and butter together. Sprinkle on top of apples.
5. Bake at 180°C for 30 minutes.

LIST OF ACRONYMS

AGEs	advanced glycation end-products
BMI	body mass index
BMR	basal metabolic rate
CAD	coronary artery disease
CHD	coronary heart disease
CLAs	conjugated linoleic acids
GERD	gastroesophageal reflux disease
GDP	gross domestic product
GHD	growth hormone deficiency
GI	glycaemic index
HDL	high-density lipoprotein
HFCS	high-fructose corn syrup
IBW	ideal body weight
IDF	International Diabetes Federation
IVF	in vitro fertilization
LDL	low-density lipoprotein
MCTs	medium-chain triglycerides
MSG	monosodium glutamate
MUFAs	monounsaturated fatty acids
PCOS	polycystic ovarian syndrome
PUFAs	polyunsaturated fatty acids

SFAs	saturated fatty acids
TFA	trans-fatty acids
USFDA	United States Food and Drug Administration
VLCDs	very low calorie diets
WC	waist circumference
WHO	World Health Organization
WHtR	waist-to-height ratio

GLOSSARY

English	Hindi
Black-eyed beans	Lobiya
Black gram	Urad dal/kala chana
Bottle gard	Doodhi/lauki/ghia
Chickpea	Safed chana
Colocasia	Arbi
Corn on the cob	Bhutta
Cottage cheese	Paneer
Cumin seeds	Jeera
Fenugreek	Methi
Fenugreek powder	Kasuri methi
Finger millet	Ragi
Gram (roasted)	Bhuna chana
Gram/pulse/chickpea flour	Besan
High-fibre rice	Samak chawal
Lemon water	Nimbu-pani
Puffed rice	Murmura
Refined flour	Maida
Roasted rice flakes	Chirwa
Semolina	Sooji/rawa

English	Hindi
Sesame seed	Til
Turmeric powder	Haldi
Unrefined sugar	Shakkar
Whole-wheat flour	Atta
Yam	Jimikand

BIBLIOGRAPHY

Assunção, M.L., H.S. Ferreira, A.F. dos Santos, C.R. Cabral Jr and T.M. Florêncio. 'Effects of Dietary Coconut Oil on the Biochemical and Anthropometric Profiles of Women Presenting Abdominal Obesity'. *Lipids* 44, no. 2 (July 2009): 593–601.

Brian Wansink. 'The Forgotten Food'. In *Mindless Eating: Why We Eat More Than We Think.* New Delhi: Hay House, 2009.

Christopher Wanjek. 'The History and Economics of Workplace Nutrition'. In *Food at Work: Workplace Solutions for Malnutrition, Obesity and Chronic Diseases.* Geneva: Publications Bureau, International Labour Office, 2005.

Enas, Enas A. and Sudesh Kannan. 'Heart Disease in Particular Populations: Cracking the Indian Paradox'. In *How to Beat the Heart Disease Epidemic among South Asians: A Prevention and Management Guide for Asian Indians and Their Doctors.* Illinois: Advanced Heart Lipid Clinic, 2005.

Fullerton-Smith, Jill. *The Truth about Food.* London: Bloomsbury, 2007.

Goodhealthindia.in. 'Obesity: Silent Killer in India'. Available online at http://goodhealthindia.in/obesity.html.

Gray, J., and B. Griffin. 'Eggs and Dietary Cholesterol—Dispelling the Myth'. *Nutrition Bulletin* 34, no. 1 (March 2009): 66–70.

Johnson, R.J., S.E. Perez-Pozo, Y.Y. Sautin, J. Manitus, L.G. Sanchez-Lozada, D.I. Feiq, M. Shafiu and others. 'Hypothesis: Could Excessive

Fructose Intake and Uric Acid Cause Type 2 Diabetes?' *Endocrine Reviews* 30, no. 1 (February 2009): 96–119.

Jonnalagadda, S.S., L. Harnack, R.H. Liu, N. McKeown, C. Seal, S. Liu and G.C. Fahey. 'Putting the Whole Grain Puzzle Together: Health Benefits Associated with Whole Grains—Summary of American Society for Nutrition 2010 Satellite Symposium'. *The Journal of Nutrition* 141, no. 5 (May 2011): 1011S–22S.

Klein S., L. Fontana, V.L. Young, A.R. Coggan, C. Kilo, B.W. Patterson and B.S. Mohammed. 'Absence of an Effect of Liposuction on Insulin Action and Risk Factors for Coronary Heart Disease'. *The New England Journal of Medicine* 350, no. 25 (June 2004): 2549–57.

Link, Lilli B. and John D. Potter. 'Raw versus Cooked Vegetables and Cancer Risk'. *Cancer Epidemiology, Biomarkers and Prevention* 13, no. 9 (September 2004): 1422–35.

Nakagawa, T., H. Hu, S. Zharikov, K.R. Tuttle, R.A. Short, O. Glushakova, X. Ouyang and others. 'A Casual Role for Uric Acid in Fructose-induced Metabolic Syndrome'. *American Journal of Physiology—Renal Physiology* 290, no. 3 (March 2006): F625–31.

Reungjui, S., C.A. Roncal, W. Mu, T.R. Srinivas, D. Sirivongs, R.J. Johnson and Nakaqawa. 'Thiazide Diuretics Exacerbate Fructose-induced Metabolic Syndrome'. *Journal of American Society of Nephrology* 18, no. 10 (October 2007): 2724–31.

Salmon, J., A. Bauman, D. Crawford, A. Timperio and N. Owen. 'The Association between Television Viewing and Overweight among Australian Adults Participating in Varying Levels of Leisure-time Physical Activity'. *International Journal of Obesity and Related Metabolic Disorders* 24, no. 5 (May 2000): 600–06.

Sicree, R., J. Shaw and P. Zimmet. 'Diabetes and Impaired Glucose Tolerance'. *IDF Diabetes Journal* 3 (2006): 15–103.

Su, L.J. and L. Arab. 'Salad and Raw Vegetable Consumption and Nutritional Status in the Population: Results from the Third National

Examination Survey'. *Journal of American Dietetic Association* 106, no. 9 (September 2006): 1394–404.

Weisell, Robert C. 'Body Mass Index as an Indicator of Obesity'. *Asia Pacific Journal of Clinical Nutrition* 11, no. 8 (December 2002): S681–84.

WHO Media Centre. 'Obesity and Overweight: Fact Sheet'. Uploaded May 2012. Available online at http://www.who.int/mediacentre/factsheets/fs311/en/.

WHO. 'Obesity: Preventing and Managing the Global Epidemic; Report of a WHO Consultation'. *WHO Technical Report Series 894* (2008): i–xii, 1–253.

ACKNOWLEDGEMENTS

During my life, many people have walked beside me and helped me along the way.

This book is thanks to all my patients. They have been a source of my learning. They have taught me what books don't teach. A special thanks to all those patients who have been generous and have shared their personal journeys of weight loss in this book.

I am deeply indebted to Dr Naresh Trehan for having faith in me and giving me the opportunity that was the stepping stone for my career. I must also acknowledge the support of Dr Peeyush Jain, Dr R.R. Kasliwal, Dr Ashok Sharma, Dr Bhavna Barmi and several friends and colleagues in the Department of Preventive Cardiology and Rehabilitation of the Escorts Heart Institute who have taught me invaluable lessons, which have helped shape my career. People who have contributed in their own special ways include Dr Ambrish Mithal, Dr Anoop Misra, Dr Alok Chopra, Dr Ashwini Chopra, Dr Archana Arya, Dr Manju Dang, Dr Navin Dang, Dr Kanak Panday and Dr Divya Parashar.

A very special thanks to my friend Chitra Narayan who initiated this book and made it possible through her hard work and efforts.

My life and career would not have been what they are without the support of the media who gave my thoughts a voice. I would like to express special thanks to all those in the media who have helped me grow, some of whom have also become close friends.

My eternal gratitude to my mentor, the late Dr M.M.S Ahuja, and all those who laid the foundation for my academic career—my principal, the late Mr M.N. Kapur, and my teachers, Ms Geeta Dudeja, Ms Kona Roy and Ms Rita Talwar, at Modern School. I would also like to thank Dr Veenu Seth, Dr Kiran Malhotra, Dr Usha Bhargava, Dr Usha Raina, Dr Bhanumati Sharma and all the other faculty members in the Foods and Nutrition Department at Lady Irwin College.

A lot of learning in my life has come about because of my wonderful family (Mehtas and Khoslas)—my brothers, brothers-in-law and sisters-in-law, my nephews Vahin, Yuv, Gautam, Saurabh, Aditya and my niece Ayesha. Our family is obsessed with good and well-presented food, constantly raising the bar for 'tasty food', and keeping me on my toes to combine health and taste. They have subconsciously contributed to this book and have inspired me. Thank you all.

My greatest joys, my two boys Karan and Dev and my husband Gagan, who have helped me to discover myself, brought out the best in me and have been my constant support, energizers and strength—thanks for your love, patience and guidance. And how can I forget our dog Dollar, my constant companion during the writing of this book and the best stress buster in the world. He is bright and youthful at 17 years of age, and exemplifies the theory that eating less is the key to longevity!

Much of what I am is thanks to my parents and parents-in-law who have taught me humility, the important values of life and how to cope and understand others' needs—especially my mother, who has always stood by me as a pillar of strength.

A heartfelt thanks to my friends, especially Kumkum and Noreen, who have been invaluable supporters and critics.

A big thank you to my partners in our health food company—Whole Foods India—in particular, Hema, Bhutto, Neerja, Tirath and Vivek who have all contributed in special ways and have made healthy food options possible, making many weight-watchers' journeys easy and enjoyable. I must also thank Ms Veena Katyal—her readiness and enthusiasm to create healthy recipes is greatly appreciated.

Finally, a heartfelt thanks to our dear Gayatri without whom I cannot ever imagine functioning—who has spent as many hours sitting by her keyboard typing out my words as I have spent writing them. She has been the strength that has driven me onwards. Always ready to work with no boundaries, she has kept me focused—letting me be when I was irritable and calming me when stressed. I hope she can rest for a while before we begin the next book. Incidentally, she is amazingly creative and a great artist! I wish her the best in life.

A sincere thanks to my staff at home and office, without whose backup I could not have managed.

I thank Penguin Books India for having the faith in me and deeply appreciate all the efforts made in making this book possible.

I would also like to thank all those who have touched my life but whose names have not been mentioned.

Finally, my best wishes to all my readers. I sincerely hope that each one of you gets some value from this book as you drop the kilos.